CASE STUDIES IN

DISCARD

MEDICAL
MICROBIOLOGY

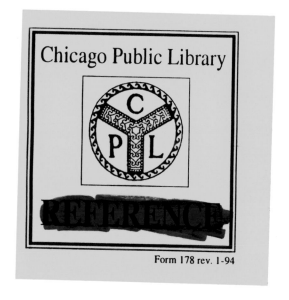

CASE STUDIES IN

MEDICAL MICROBIOLOGY

Cedric A Mims BSc MD FRCPath
Emeritus Professor
Department of Microbiology
Guy's Hospital Medical School
London, UK

Gillian Urwin MSc MBBS MRCPath
Lecturer
Department of Medical Microbiology
The London Hospital Medical College
London, UK

Mark A Zuckerman BSc(Hons) MSc MRCP MRCPath
Clinical Lecturer/Honorary Senior Registrar
Department of Medical Microbiology
University College London Medical School
London, UK

M Mosby

Copyright © 1994 Times Mirror International Publishers Limited
Published in 1994 by Mosby–Wolfe, an imprint of Times Mirror International Publishers Limited
Printed by Grafos S.A. Arte sobre papel, Barcelona, Spain
ISBN 0 7234 2051 3

For full details of all Times Mirror International Publishers Ltd. titles please write to Times Mirror International
Publishers Ltd., Lynton House, 7–12 Tavistock Square, London WC1H 9LB, England.

A CIP catalogue record for this book is available from the British Library.

REFACE

The fifty case histories in this book are a companion to the *Medical Microbiology* textbook to which each case is cross referenced.

This book is primarily for undergraduate students and the answers should be supplemented by the relevant sections of the main text. Each case has an accompanying case revision box in which additional notes can be included.

We have aimed to give a flavour of the clinical presentation, differential diagnosis, laboratory tests and aspects of control of infection which are critical in the everyday management of patients with infectious diseases.

CKNOWLEDGEMENTS

We thank Dr Rosemary Williams, Dr Melinda Tenant-Flowers, Dr Begoña Bovill, Dr Nick Banatvala, Dr Tanya Levine, and Moya Briggs for helpful advice.

Finally we are grateful to our publishers, Dr Tracy Cooper and Linda Kull.

NORMAL VALUES, ABBREVIATIONS, AND DEFINITIONS

NORMAL RANGES (ADULTS)		
Investigation		
Blood tests		
	Males	**Females**
Haemoglobin (Hb)	13.0–18.0 g/dl	11.5–16.5 g/dl
White cell count (WCC)	4.0–11.0 x10^9/l	
Platelets	150–440 x10^9/l	
Erythrocyte Sedimentation Rate (ESR)	0–6 mm/hr (under 60 years of age)	
Potassium	3.5–5.0 mmol/l	
Sodium	135–145 mmol/l	
Glucose (fasting)	<5.5 mmol/l	
Urea	2.5–6.7 mmol/l	
Creatinine	70–150 micromol/l	
Alkaline phosphatase (ALP)	30–300 IU/l	
Alanine amino transferase (ALT)	5–35 IU/l	
Aspartate amino transferase (AST)	5–35 IU/l	
Bilirubin	3–17 micromol/l	
Cerebrospinal fluid (CSF)		
White cells	0–5 lymphocytes /mm^3	
Glucose	2.8–3.9 mmol/l	
Protein	0.15–0.45 g/l	

ABBREVIATIONS AND DEFINITIONS

A&E	Accident and emergency department / Emergency room
ALP	Alkaline phosphatase
ALT	Alanine amino transferase
AST	Aspartate amino transferase
CFT	Complement Fixation Test
CSF	Cerebrospinal fluid
ELISA	Enzyme Linked ImmunoSorbent Assay
ITU	Intensive therapy unit / intensive care unit

Dyspnoea	difficulty breathing
Dyspareunia	painful sexual intercourse
Dysuria	painful micturition
Epistaxis	nose bleed
Fomites	contaminated objects
Photophobia	light sensitivity
Tachycardia	rapid pulse rate
Tachypnoea	rapid respiratory rate

CONTENTS

1 UPPER RESPIRATORY TRACT INFECTIONS

CASE 1

An 18-month-old girl presents to the Accident & Emergency Dept. (A&E) in the early hours of the morning having woken up screaming with a fever. Her parents are unable to console her. She has a three-day history of cold and snuffles.

On examination, she is flushed and irritable, and her ear drums are bright red and bulging.

Questions
1 What is the diagnosis?
2 What are the most likely pathogens?
3 How would you treat her?
4 What are the possible complications of this condition?

Notes for revision

see Mims 20.7

Your answers

Case 1

1 **Diagnosis**

2 **Most likely pathogens**

3 **Treatment**

4 **Possible complications**

CASE 2

A previously healthy two-year-old boy presents with a six-hour history of fever and difficulty in swallowing. His mother has noticed that his breathing has become increasingly harsh. Systematic enquiry reveals that he received only one dose of the usual childhood vaccinations because the family had moved when he was four months old and he was lost to follow up. There is no family history of note. He has one older sibling who is well.

On examination he is febrile and obviously distressed. His breathing is harsh, with a marked inspiratory stridor. His ears are normal and his chest is clear. The results of initial investigations are shown in Fig.1.1.

FIG. 1.1 RESULTS OF INITIAL INVESTIGATIONS	
Investigation	**Result**
Haemoglobin	16 g/dl
White cell count	14 x 10^9/l with 90% neutrophils
Urea and electrolytes	Normal
Chest radiograph	Normal

Questions
1 What is the differential diagnosis?
2 What other investigations would be helpful?
3 What is the pathogen responsible for this condition, and how would you treat the infection?

see Mims 20.7

Your answers

Case 2

1 **Differential diagnosis**

2 **Other investigations**

3 **Pathogen responsible and treatment**

CASE 1

Answers

1 Diagnosis
Acute otitis media.

2 Most likely pathogens
Haemophilus influenzae and *Streptococcus pneumoniae* are the most common pathogens. Less commonly *Moraxella catarrhalis*, Group A beta haemolytic streptococci, and *Staphylococcus aureus* are implicated. Acute otitis media often follows a viral upper respiratory tract infection. Congestion of the eustachian tubes results in fluid stasis within the middle ear and secondary bacterial infection. The pressure building up within the anatomical constraints of the middle ear causes pain, and may lead to perforation of the tympanic membrane, with a discharge of pus.

3 Treatment
Treatment should involve systemic antibiotics, usually oral unless the child is vomiting. Options include amoxycillin either alone or in combination with a beta lactamase inhibitor such as clavulanic acid to cover the increasing proportion of *H. influenzae* that are beta lactamase positive. Alternatives include orally active second and third generation cephalosporins. Penicillin-allergic patients should be given cotrimoxazole or a new macrolide with increased activity against *H. influenzae*.

4 Possible complications
Complications include acute mastoiditis, which is rare since the advent of antibiotic therapy, and recurrent infections leading to chronic exudative otitis media (glue ear), which is a much more common problem.

....

CASE 2

Answers

1 Differential diagnosis?
The differential diagnosis should include the following.
- Acute epiglottitis.
- Respiratory obstruction due to an inhaled foreign body.
- Croup.

2 Other investigations
- Blood culture would identify any pathogen responsible for septicaemia.
- A radiograph of the epiglottic region would identify a swollen epiglottis. It may help identify any foreign bodies. Such cases are medical emergencies as tracheal obstruction may occur. An anaesthetist is required to assist in intubation.

    It is most important in a suspected case of epiglottitis NOT to perform an examination of the throat and pharynx as this may cause the epiglottis to obstruct the trachea.

3 Pathogen responsible and treatment
Haemophilus influenzae capsular type b (Hib) is responsible for the majority of cases of epiglottitis. Antibiotics suitable for treatment include third generation cephalosporins such as cefotaxime and ceftriaxone. It may be necessary to intubate and ventilate the patient if there is severe respiratory distress.

    With the increasing use of immunisation against Hib, the invasive diseases it causes such as meningitis, pneumonia, and epiglottitis will become rare. However, this pathogen must not be forgotten in the unimmunised population, including immigrants from countries where Hib immunisation is not routine.

Notes for revision

see Mims 21.1–21.4

CASE 3

A 42-year-old homosexual man with acquired immunodeficiency syndrome (AIDS), complains of blurred vision. He has noticed that he has floaters and a visual field loss, which he describes as black patches in his vision. His last CD4 count was very low at 20 cells/mm^3 and he has been admitted to hospital for treatment of *Pneumocystis carinii* pneumonia and Kaposi's sarcoma.

Fundoscopy reveals areas of white infiltrates and haemorrhages consistent with a diagnosis of retinitis. Examination of his visual fields reveals a single scotoma (a blind spot) in the inferotemporal part of his retina.

Questions

1 What infections are associated with a choroidoretinitis?
2 How would you make the diagnosis?
3 How would you treat a patient with CMV retinitis?

Notes for revision

Your answers

1 Infections associated with a choroidoretinitis?

2 How would you make the diagnosis?

3 Treatment for CMV retinitis

CASE 3

Answers

1 Infections associated with a choroidoretinitis?

Cytomegalovirus (CMV), *Toxoplasma gondii*, *Toxocara* (*canis* or *catis*), *Mycobacterium tuberculosis*, or acute retinal necrosis, which is thought to be associated with varicella zoster virus.

2 How would you make the diagnosis?

The diagnosis is almost invariably clinical and is made with the assistance of an ophthalmologist. In such a patient it can sometimes be difficult to differentiate between *Toxoplasma* and CMV. CMV retinitis sometimes has a classical appearance referred to as tomato ketchup and cottage cheese! Serology may be helpful in the diagnosis of *Toxoplasma* infection.

In addition, in certain centres vitreous fluid from the affected eye can be collected. Detection of CMV DNA in this sample can be performed using a nested polymerase chain reaction approach involving two sets of primers, one set internal to the other, which increases the sensitivity of the test.

3 Treatment for CMV retinitis

Commence with a treatment course of intravenous ganciclovir while monitoring the haemoglobin, white cell count, and platelet count because this antiviral drug is myelosuppressive. If bone marrow suppression occurs an alternative drug is foscarnet (which is nephrotoxic).

It is best to site permanent intravenous access as this patient will need maintenance therapy with either of these drugs together with regular ophthalmological follow up to detect and prevent reactivation.

Notes for revision

LOWER RESPIRATORY TRACT INFECTIONS

CASE 4

see Mims 22.5–22.8

A 30-year-old man presents with a ten-day history of tiredness, headache, fever, and dry cough. He smokes 20 cigarettes a day, his past medical history is unremarkable, and there is nothing else of note on systems review.

Relevant findings on examination include a temperature of 38°C, dyspnoea, and a skin rash consistent with erythema multiforme. Auscultation of his chest reveals a few scattered crepitations and is otherwise unremarkable. The results of investigations are shown in Fig. 3.1.

FIG. 3.1 RESULTS OF INVESTIGATIONS

Investigation	Result
Haemoglobin	10 g/dl
White cell count	6×10^9/l
Erythrocyte sedimentation rate	45 mm/hr
Urea and electrolytes	Normal
Chest radiograph	Patchy shadowing

Questions

1 What is the differential diagnosis?
2 Which questions particularly relevant to this differential diagnosis have not been asked?
3 What further investigations would you perform?
4 The results of some of these investigations are given in Fig. 3.2. What is the diagnosis?

FIG. 3.2 RESULTS OF FURTHER INVESTIGATIONS

Investigation	Result
Mycoplasma particle agglutination test titre	1024
Mycoplasma CFT acute serum titre	160
Mycoplasma CFT convalescent serum titre	2560
Cold agglutinins	Positive

5 How would you treat this patient?

Notes for revision

Your answers

1 Differential diagnosis

2 Other questions particularly relevant to the differential diagnosis to ask

3 Further investigations

4 Diagnosis

5 Treatment

CASE 4

Answers

1 Differential diagnosis

This case is suggestive of an atypical pneumonia. Causes are:

- Chlamydial infections (e.g. *Chlamydia pneumoniae* (also referred to as TWAR), *Chlamydia psittaci*).
- *Mycoplasma pneumoniae*.
- *Legionella pneumophila*.
- *Coxiella burnetii* (Q fever).

2 Other questions particularly relevant to the differential diagnosis to ask

- What is your occupation?
- Have you travelled recently?
- Do you have any pets at home or any hobbies?

These questions are always an important part of the history, but may be especially relevant with regard to *Chlamydia psittaci* (contact with infected birds), *Legionella pneumophila* (air conditioning systems), and *Coxiella burnetii*/Q fever (contact with infected sheep/cattle).

3 Further investigations

Serology

- **To detect *Mycoplasma pneumoniae*** Particle agglutination test (IgM and IgG) and complement fixation test (CFT) on paired acute and convalescent sera collected 10–14 days apart, or test the acute serum specimen taken at least ten days after the illness. The haematology laboratory should also test for the presence of cold agglutinins.
- **To detect *Chlamydia group*** Microimmunofluorescence for type-specific IgM/IgG or ELISA, and CFT on paired acute and convalescent sera collected 10–14 days apart, or test the acute serum taken at least ten days after the illness. The CFT uses the chlamydial group-specific antigen.
- **To detect *Legionella pneumophila*** Rapid MicroAgglutination Test (RMAT) to detect the presence of antibody.
- **To detect *Coxiella burnetii*** CFT of paired acute and convalescent sera collected 10–14 days apart, or test the acute serum specimen taken at least ten days after the illness. Phase 1 antibody is detected in chronic Q fever infection. Phase 2 antibody is detected in acute and chronic Q fever infection.

Culture for *Chlamydia*, *Mycoplasma*, and *Legionella* may be attempted, depending on available laboratory facilities.

4 Diagnosis

Mycoplasma pneumoniae infection on the basis of a four-fold rise in CFT, a positive agglutination test titre having diluted the serum 1 in 1024, and positive cold agglutinins.

5 Treatment

The antibiotics of choice are erythromycin or tetracycline.

Notes for revision

CASE 5

see Mims 22.1

An eight-month-old girl presents with a three-week history of a cough. She initially had a runny nose and her mother thought she had a viral infection. However, the cough appears to be worsening, particularly at night. It often comes in spasms and she frequently vomits after coughing. The mother, who is a teacher, also has a mild cough and has taken the past two weeks off work, both to nurse the child and because she was feeling unwell herself.

On examination, the child appears mildly dehydrated but not distressed. Her chest is clear and her abdominal examination is normal.

Questions

1 What important points have been omitted from the history?
2 What are the possible infectious causes of this girl's cough?
3 What are the complications of infection?
4 What preventive measures are available to control this disease?

Notes for revision

Your answers

1 Important point omitted from the history

2 Possible infectious causes of this girl's cough

3 Complications of infection

4 Preventive measures available to control this disease

CASE 5

Answers

1 Important points omitted from history

A past medical history, family history of disease and vaccination history should be taken. The child has been previously well, but was not immunised with the normal childhood vaccinations as there was a family history of epilepsy in the maternal uncle.

2 Possible infectious causes of this girl's cough

This child's cough could be due to a viral infection, such as respiratory syncytial virus, influenza, parainfluenza or adenovirus. However, the long history of the spasms of coughing associated with vomiting in a child who has not been immunised is often a symptom of *Bordetella pertussis* (whooping cough) infection. A pernasal swab should be taken and cultured on *Bordetella* selective media. If a full blood count is performed, a marked lymphocytosis is often seen.

Adults may be infected with *B.pertussis*, and the mother's infection may be due to this organism.

3 Complications of infection

The complications of pertussis can be serious and it is associated with substantial morbidity and mortality. These include bronchopneumonia, which may be in part due to secondary infection with organisms such as *Haemophilus influenzae*; atelectasis, which may result in bronchiectasis; and convulsions after a severe paroxysm of coughing may lead to intracerebral haemorrhage.

The pressure of paroxysmal coughing may cause conjunctival haemorrhage and epistaxis. A frenal ulcer may appear on the tongue in the early stages of disease.

4 Prevention

Immunisation is recommended for all children against pertussis unless there is a specific contraindication. There is much debate about the association of pertussis immunisation and neurological damage. One national encephalopathy study has followed up cases and has not shown convincing evidence that there is an association with immunisation. Certainly the risk of cerebral damage from the disease is much greater than that of the immunisation.

Pertussis immunisation is contraindicated in patients where there is evidence of a progressive neurological deficit, or a family history of neurological disease in a first degree relative.

CASE 6

An 18-year-old ballet dancer with long-standing insulin-dependent mellitus (IDDM) is admitted to hospital because her diabetes has become difficult to control; she is hyperglycaemic and has become extremely unwell. She had an initial history of a fever of sudden onset with a high temperature of 40°C, headache, aching muscles and joints, and a sore throat. After about a week some of her symptoms resolved, but she started to have rigors and a cough productive of dirty green sputum.

On examination she is tachypnoeic and dyspnoeic and is unable to give a history. She has a temperature of 40°C, her pulse is 100 beats/min and regular, and her blood pressure 90/60 mm Hg. Examination of her respiratory system reveals that her trachea is central and a few wheezes and crackles are heard on auscultation. The results of investigations are shown in Fig. 3.3.

FIG. 3.3 RESULTS OF INVESTIGATIONS	
Investigation	Result
Haemoglobin	13 g/dl
White cell count	24×10^9/l with 70% neutrophils
Platelets	250×10^9/l
Glucose	45 mmol/l
Urea	30 mmol/l
Chest radiograph	Multiple opacities consistent with lung abscesses

Questions

1 What other investigations would you perform?
2 What is the most likely initial diagnosis and final diagnosis?
3 How would you manage her?
4 What would be your advice about prophylaxis against viral respiratory tract infections?

Notes for revision

see Mims 22.10–22.13

Your answers

1 Other investigations

2 Most likely initial diagnosis and final diagnosis

3 Management

4 Advice about prophylaxis against viral respiratory tract infections

CASE 6

Answers

1 **Other investigations**
   - Arterial blood gas analysis.
   - Blood cultures: *Staphylococcus aureus* was grown from blood cultures after 24 hours.
   - Sputum culture: *Staph. aureus* was grown from a sputum culture.
   - Antibiotic sensitivity testing.
   - Serum complement fixation tests for influenza A, influenza B, mycoplasma, chlamydia, *Coxiella burnetii* . These gave the following results: influenza A (1280), influenza B (40), mycoplasma (<40), chlamydia (<40), *Coxiella burnetii* (<40).

2 **Most likely initial diagnosis and final diagnosis**
   Acute influenza A viral infection complicated by a *Staph. aureus* septicaemia with seeding to the lungs resulting in abscess formation.

3 **Management**
   - Rehydrate with intravenous fluids and stabilise her diabetes using an insulin pump on a sliding scale.
   - Give intravenous antibiotics (e.g. flucloxacillin if the *Staph. aureus* is sensitive to this antibiotic).
   - Arrange physiotherapy for when she is less acutely unwell
   - Oxygen (the oxygen concentration delivered will be determined by the results of the arterial blood gas analysis).
   - Follow up chest radiograph.

4 **Advice about prophylaxis against viral respiratory tract infections**
   It is generally recommended that people with IDDM should be offered influenza immunisation annually.

Notes for revision

CASE 7

see Mims 22.2–22.4

A 10-month-old baby boy is brought in to hospital by his mother with a fever, coryza, dry cough, and shortness of breath. He has become more restless with a worsening cough over the past day. There is no relevant past medical history and he is up to date with his immunisation schedule.

On examination he is unwell with an elevated respiratory rate, nasal flaring, chest wall retraction, and a temperature of 38°C. Auscultation of his chest reveals generalised wheezing. The results of investigations are shown in Fig. 3.4. A diagnosis of acute bronchiolitis is made.

FIG. 3.4 RESULTS OF INVESTIGATIONS	
Investigation	**Result**
Full blood count	Normal
Urea and electrolytes	Normal
Chest radiograph	Hyperinflated lung fields with areas of atelectasis

Questions

1 What are the most likely viral causes of acute bronchiolitis?
2 What further investigations would you perform?
3 The child's condition worsens during the night. What would be your further management?
4 What control of infection measures would you instigate?

Your answers

1 **Most likely viral causes of acute bronchiolitis**

2 **Further investigations**

3 **Further management**

4 **Control of infection measures**

Notes for revision

CASE 7

Answers

1 Most likely viral causes of acute bronchiolitis

Respiratory synctial virus (RSV), parainfluenza types 1–3, adenoviruses, and influenza viral infections.

2 Further investigations

A nasopharyngeal aspirate should be collected. A rapid viral diagnosis using immunofluorescence to detect viral antigen in infected nasopharyngeal epithelial cells may be made. The time taken from specimen preparation to reading the result is approximately three hours. RSV is detected by immunofluorescence.

3 Further management

- Supportive care with oxygen.
- Arterial blood gas analysis.
- Consider treating with the antiviral drug ribavirin using the recommendations of the American Academy of Paediatricians. Ribavirin is given by a small particle aerosol generator in an intensive care unit setting. Side-effects include precipitation of the drug in ventilator tubes and development of rashes in attending members of staff.

4 Control of infection measures

RSV may be spread by droplet/aerosol and by fomites. Source isolation should therefore be instituted; handwashing, and gloves and masks are recommended for any members of staff looking after the patient.

Notes for revision

CASE 8

see Mims 22.5–22.8

A 41-year-old Nigerian man presents with a one-day history of high fever with rigors and pleuritic chest pain. He has a cough and is producing green blood-flecked sputum. He is known to have sickle cell trait.

On examination he appears unwell and has rigors. His temperature is 40°C. He has a tender chest wall, an increased respiratory rate, and oral herpetic lesions. His pulse rate is 120 beats/min, and blood pressure is 90/50 mm Hg. On auscultation of his chest he is noted to have bronchial breathing and coarse crackles in the region of the right lower lobe. The results of investigations are shown in Fig. 3.5.

FIG. 3.5 RESULTS OF INVESTIGATIONS	
Investigation	**Result**
Haemoglobin	13 g/dl
White cell count	22×10^9/l with 90% neutrophils
Chest radiograph	Right lower lobe pneumonia

Questions

1 What is the diagnosis and how would you treat this infection?
2 What is the major predisposing factor for infection in this man and how can recurrences of this infection be prevented?

Notes for revision

Your answers

Case 2

1 **Diagnosis and treatment**

2 **Major predisposing factor for infection in this man and how recurrences of this infection can be prevented**

CASE 8

Answers

1 Diagnosis and treatment

The diagnosis is lobar pneumonia due to *Streptococcus pneumoniae*. The drug of choice for the treatment of pneumococcal infections is benzylpenicillin. Penicillin resistance has been described in many countries and can cause problems in treating pneumococcal infections. For pneumonia due to *S. pneumoniae* with reduced susceptibility to benzylpenicillin, infections may respond to high-dose benzylpenicillin. However, in cases of meningitis with this pathogen, a cephalosporin such as cefotaxime or ceftriaxone should be used. A smaller number of cases of *S. pneumoniae* that are resistant to penicillin have been reported. In all infections with such organisms, cefotaxime or ceftriaxone should be used.

Treatment of patients who are allergic to penicillin is more problematic: chloramphenicol, glycopeptide antibiotics (e.g. vancomycin, teicoplanin), and a macrolide antibiotic such as erythromycin can be used.

2 Major predisposing factor for infection in this man and how recurrences of this infection can be prevented

People with a non-functioning spleen are particularly susceptible to pneumococcal infection. The risk of acquiring pneumococcal disease can be reduced by giving a polysaccharide pneumococcal vaccine or oral penicillin in low doses for life. The vaccine is most effective in people in whom the spleen is present. Therefore if the spleen is removed electively, the vaccine should be given before splenectomy. Low-dose penicillin may be a more appropriate therapy to prevent pneumococcal infection in people with sickle cell disease who undergo autosplenectomy.

CASE 9

A 32-year-old Indian male who has been resident in the UK for six months presents to the chest clinic with a three-month history of fatigue, weight loss, fever, and night sweats. He has a cough which is worsening and has recently produced blood-stained sputum. He is breathless on exertion and smokes 10 cigarettes a day. He has no past medical history of note.

On examination, he is thin and wasted. His temperature is 37.8°C, and he is dyspnoeic at rest. Chest auscultation is consistent with right apical consolidation. The results of investigations are shown in Fig. 3.6.

FIG. 3.6 RESULTS OF INVESTIGATIONS	
Investigation	**Result**
Haemoglobin	11 g/dl (normochromic normocytic film)
White cell count	14 x10^9/l with 70% neutrophils
Erythrocyte sedimentation rate	80 mm/hr
Chest radiograph	Right apical shadowing

Questions

1 What is the most likely infectious cause of this man's symptoms?
2 How is this infection diagnosed?
3 What antimicrobial therapy is indicated?
4 What control of infection measures are necessary if he is admitted to the ward?

Notes for revision

see Mims 22.14–22.17

Your answers

1 **Most likely infectious cause**

2 **How this infection is diagnosed**

3 **Antimicrobial therapy**

4 **Control of infection measures**

CASE 9

Answers

1 Most likely infectious cause

The history of weight loss, night sweats, and cough in an immigrant from Asia strongly suggests *Mycobacterium tuberculosis* infection.

2 How this infection is diagnosed

Demonstration of acid-fast rods in the sputum using either Ziehl-Neelsen or auramine stains gives a rapid diagnosis of tuberculosis. Culture of *Mycobacteria* is a lengthy procedure and can take several months.

3 Antimicrobial therapy

Mycobacterium tuberculosis infections require treatment with multiple antimicrobial agents to minimise the risk of the development of resistance while the patient is being treated. Current recommendations depend on the prevalence of resistant isolates; in pulmonary tuberculosis in which the organism is fully susceptible, regimes should include rifampicin and isoniazid, with a third antituberculous drug.

Triple therapy is continued for a period of two months, and then isoniazid and rifampicin are continued for a total of nine months. Shorter course therapy is currently the subject of some research.

4 Control of infection measures

Patients with open tuberculosis should be nursed in a side room in source isolation for the first two weeks of therapy. Source isolation reduces the risk of spread of *Mycobacterium tuberculosis* to other patients and staff members. This is a notifiable disease and contact tracing together with follow up of all contacts must be instituted immediately.

Notes for revision

CASE 10

see Mims Chapter 23

An eight-month-old boy presents to A&E in the early hours of the morning with a 24-hour history of being irritable, off his feeds, and not sleeping. Over the previous six hours he has developed a temperature and has started vomiting. He has no diarrhoea.

On examination he is irritable and difficult to examine. He is mildly dehydrated, and his temperature is 38°C. His fontanelle is not raised and there are no focal neurological signs. Examination of his ears, nose, and throat is normal, and examination of his chest, cardiovascular system, and abdomen is unremarkable.

He lives with his mother and two older siblings and has a complete vaccination history.

Questions

1 What investigations would you request in A&E?
2 How would you manage this boy?
3 What follow up would you plan?

Your answers

1 Investigations in casualty

2 Management

3 Follow up

Notes for revision

CASE 10

Answers

1 **Investigations in A&E**

The following investigations were performed:

- A clean catch specimen of urine: urine microscopy revealed more than 1000 white blood cells /mm^3, with many bacteria present.
- Full blood count: haemoglobin was 15 g/l, white cell count 17×10^9/l.
- Urea and electrolytes: urea 5.6 mmol/l, creatinine 72 mmol/l, potassium 4.2 mmol/l, and sodium 136 mmol/l.

2 **Management**

He has a urinary tract infection with mild dehydration. He should be admitted to hospital and fed by nasogastric tube if he continues to vomit. He may need intravenous fluids. Antibiotics should be given and amended if necessary on the basis of the urine culture results.

3 **Follow up**

Children often improve rapidly and can be discharged after a few days. However, it is necessary to investigate renal function and assess any renal scarring with scans which assess both renal function and anatomy. A micturating cystogram will identify vesico-ureteric reflux.

CASE 11

An eight-month pregnant 22-year-old teacher presents to her doctor with a 48-hour history of dysuria and lower abdominal pain. This is her first pregnancy, and it has previously been unremarkable.

On examination she is apyrexial and her uterus is normal size for dates. There is some lower abdominal tenderness, but her renal angles are not tender. A dipstix test of her urine in the surgery reveals the presence of protein, but no glucose or blood. Her urine is sent for culture in the laboratory and grows more than 10^5 coliforms/mm^3.

Questions?

1 What antimicrobials are appropriate for use in pregnancy?
2 Why is urine screened for infection in pregnancy?

CASE 12

A 70-year-old retired army officer is referred by his doctor with acute retention of urine. He has been having increasing difficulty passing urine over the previous week. For a while he has noticed post-micturition dribbling, and that his stream is very weak.

On examination he is in obvious distress and has a distended bladder up to his umbilicus.

Questions

1 What is the most likely underlying cause of this man's acute retention?
2 What is the immediate and more long term management?

Notes for revision

see Mims Chapter 23

Your answers

Case 11

1 Antimicrobials appropriate for use in pregnancy

2 Why urine is screened for infection in pregnancy

Case 12

1 Most likely underlying cause

2 Immediate and more long term management

CASE 11

Answers

1 **Antimicrobials appropriate for use in pregnancy**

It may be possible to treat a simple urinary tract infection with a urinary sterilising agent such as nitrofurantoin. Ampicillin is a suitable first-line antibiotic in areas where there is a low prevalence of resistant *Escherichia coli*. Where the prevalence of resistance is high, it may be necessary to use an oral cephalosporin. If the patient is unwell and requires parenteral antibiotics, an injectable cephalosporin can be given.

2 **Why urine is screened for infection in pregnancy**

Pregnant women have an increased risk of developing a urinary tract infection because the ureters dilate under the action of progesterone. This allows the urine to remain static and infection to ascend from the bladder. In the early stages of infection the patient may be asymptomatic, hence the need to screen the urine for the presence of infection. The risk of pyelonephritis is greater in the pregnant woman with a positive urine culture. Both urinary tract infection and pyelonephritis may cause septicaemia, which may result in premature labour. It is therefore necessary to identify and treat urinary tract infections in pregnancy promptly.

CASE 12

Answers

1 **Most likely underlying cause**

He has bladder neck obstruction. The most likely cause in his case is benign prostatic hypertrophy. The most likely precipitant of the retention is a urinary tract infection. A mid-stream urine examination (MSU) reveals more than 10^5 coliforms /mm^3, which are sensitive to ampicillin.

2 **Immediate and more long term management**

It is necessary to relieve his acute retention immediately by passing a urethral catheter. Care must be taken to ensure that this is performed under sterile conditions and prophylaxis with an intravenous antibiotic, to which the organism is sensitive, should be given to prevent a septicaemia which may result from this procedure. Occasionally it is not possible to pass a urethral catheter because the bladder neck is tight. A suprapubic catheter may need to be inserted. Once the acute problem has settled and the infection has been treated, it is usually necessary to proceed to prostatectomy.

Notes for revision

SEXUALLY TRANSMITTED DISEASES

CASE 13

see Mims 24.11–24.13

A 29-year-old business executive presents with an offensive smelling vaginal discharge, dyspareunia and dysuria. On examination the vaginal mucosa is inflamed and a discharge is seen.

Questions

1 What are the microbiological causes of a vaginal discharge?
2 A vaginal swab is collected. What laboratory investigations would you perform on receipt of the specimen?
3 What treatment and advice would you give?

Your answers

1 Microbiological causes of a vaginal discharge

2 Laboratory investigations of a vaginal swab

3 Treatment and advice

Notes for revision

CASE 13

Answers

1 Microbiological causes of a vaginal discharge
- *Candida albicans.*
- *Trichomonas vaginalis.*
- Anaerobic vaginosis.
- *Neisseria gonorrhoeae.*
- *Chlamydia trachomatis.*
- Cervical herpes simplex virus (HSV infection).
- More rarely, foreign body-associated infections (i.e. *Staphylococcus aureus*).

2 Laboratory investigations of a vaginal swab
- Microscopy (wet preparation to look for budding yeasts and motile trichomonads).
- Gram stain and wet preparation for clue cells which are indicative of anaerobic vaginosis, and for yeasts.
- Direct culture on Sabouraud's selective medium for fungi.
- Direct culture on a VCNT plate, which contains the antibiotics vancomycin, colistin, neomycin, and trimethoprim. This suppresses the normal vaginal flora and assists the isolation of *N. gonorrhoeae*.
- Direct culture on media selective for *N. gonorrhoeae*, anaerobes and fungi.

The laboratory informs you that motile *Trichomonas vaginalis* has been seen.

3 Treatment and advice

The treatment of choice is metronidazole, and the patient should be advised to avoid sexual intercourse until the infection is cleared and that her sexual partner will also need a course of treatment. The combination of metronidazole and alcohol often leads to facial flushing due to an aldehyde effect, and so alcohol should be avoided while on treatment. A follow-up appointment with repeat microscopy and culture should be arranged. A serum sample should be tested for syphilis serology as part of the management of a patient with a sexually transmitted disease, together with health advice and counselling.

Notes for revision

CASE 14

see Mims 24.14–24.21

A 24-year-old art critic presents with a fever, dry cough, and shortness of breath for ten days, which have been getting worse. She seems very anxious, but otherwise nothing can be found either in the medical history or on physical examination. A blood sample is collected for an atypical pneumonia screen and her doctor gives her amoxycillin and erythromycin.

Five days later she feels much worse and calls her doctor, who arranges for her admission to hospital. The results of the blood tests taken after she had been ill for 10 days are shown in Fig. 5.1.

She later admits to weight loss and night sweats, and says that she has been worried because four years ago she had intimate contact over a few months with a boyfriend who was later diagnosed as HIV-1 (human immunodeficiency virus) seropositive. On examination the relevant findings are a temperature of 37.8°C, dyspnoea, and tachypnoea. There are no other findings in the respiratory system. A chest radiograph shows bilateral shadowing and a ground-glass appearance, sparing the upper zones. After appropriate counselling she consents to an HIV antibody screening test.

FIG. 5.1 RESULTS OF INVESTIGATIONS

Investigation	Result
Haemoglobin	13 g/dl
White cell count	2.3×10^9/l
Mycoplasma latex agglutination test	<8
Complement fixation test for antibodies to:	
Chlamydia group	<40
Influenza A and B	<40
Adenoviruses	<40
Mycoplasma pneumoniae	<40
Coxiella burnetii	<40

Questions

1 What is the most likely diagnosis?
2 What further investigations would you perform?
3 How would you manage her?
4 She improves over the next two weeks. What is her prognosis and how would you follow her up?

Notes for revision

Your answers

1 Most likely diagnosis

2 Further investigations

3 Management

4 Prognosis and follow up

CASE 14

Answers

1 Most likely diagnosis

Pneumocystis carinii pneumonia (PCP) in a person with HIV-1 infection.

2 Further investigations

- Arterial blood gas analysis.
- Induced sputum or bronchoscopy and bronchoalveolar lavage for PCP examination.
- HIV 1 and 2 antibody screening assay: this is positive and therefore a further confirmatory test is performed and demonstrates the presence of antibody to HIV-1. In addition, *Pneumocystis* cysts are seen on cytology. .

3 Management

The diagnosis should be discussed sensitively with her and a further serum specimen collected to confirm the diagnosis. A second specimen should always be retested to ensure that no errors in the collection, labelling of the specimen, dispatch, or handling of the specimen in the laboratory have occurred. The laboratory should have tested both the serum from the original specimen and repeat the test on any remaining serum in the original tube containing the blood clot.

First-line treatment for PCP, which would have already been started on clinical suspicion, generally comprises oxygen and cotrimoxazole, and in severe cases methylprednisolone. If she develops an allergy to the sulpha containing drugs such as cotrimoxazole, intravenous pentamidine treatment should be instituted. Clinicians will be guided by the clinical signs and symptoms as well as the results of the blood gas analysis.

4 Prognosis and follow up

She has an AIDS defining diagnosis (i.e. PCP) and her prognosis in terms of survival duration is variable. Baseline CD4 counts and a p24 antigen test would be performed as would a syphilis and viral hepatitis screen.

Regular PCP prophylaxis with cotrimoxazole should be instituted and she should be followed up regularly. She should be monitored clinically, and CD4 counts should be repeated at regular intervals. A decision about whether to start antiretroviral treatment should be discussed.

Other issues include a discussion regarding her partner and HIV testing, safe sex, and if she has or is planning to have children. Counselling about the wider aspects and implications of her diagnosis with a health advisor should be arranged.

CASE 15

see Mims 24.6–24.8

A 22-year-old estate agent returns home after a holiday to Turkey with a three-day history of dysuria and a purulent urethral discharge.

Questions

1 What is the diagnosis?
2 What investigations would you perform?
3 What is the presumptive diagnosis and how would it be established?
4 How would you manage him?

Your answers

1 Diagnosis

2 Investigations

3 Presumptive diagnosis and how it would be established

4 Management

Notes for revision

CASE 15

Answers

1 Diagnosis

The diagnosis is urethritis, which can be:

- specific (e.g. due to *Neisseria gonorrhoeae*).
- nonspecific (i.e. caused primarily by *Chlamydia trachomatis*, but also by *Ureaplasma urealyticum* or other microorganisms).

2 Investigations

- Direct smear and culture of the material collected from the urethral discharge or a urethral swab. The laboratory informs you that the direct smear contains numerous Gram-negative intracellular diplococci in the pus cells.
- Enzyme-linked immunosorbent assay (ELISA) to detect chlamydial antigen, which may be confirmed by microimmunofluorescence testing. In addition, chlamydial culture may be available in certain laboratories using McCoy tissue culture cells.

3 Presumptive diagnosis and how it would be established

The diagnosis is a *Neisseria gonorrhoeae* infection. It is established using the following methods.

- Culture on a selective medium.
- Oxidase reaction, which would be positive.
- Sugar fermentation tests. There is acid production from glucose, but not from maltose, lactose or sucrose.
- Agglutination test to confirm the identity of *N. gonorrhoeae*.
- Antibiotic sensitivity tests.

4 Management

- Antibiotic choice is dependent on knowing the antibiotic susceptibility of the organism in the country in which the infection was acquired. Treat with penicillin if the organism is a fully sensitive strain. Penicillin is the first line drug, although in many countries there is a high prevalence of penicillin-resistant gonococcal strains and alternative antibiotics are needed. In addition, doxycycline treatment is often given as chlamydial infections often complicate gonorrhoea.
- Follow up with repeat cultures.
- Contact tracing and treat the contacts to control the spread of the infection.

CASE 16

see Mims 24.1–24.5

A 50-year-old long distance truck driver is seen by his doctor complaining of shooting pains in his legs, altered sensation in his feet, and difficulty walking. He has not had a medical examination for years and has only made an appointment because he has found that he cannot feel the clutch, brake, and accelerator pedals in his truck properly. In his past medical history he had been told that he might have syphilis after developing a painless ulcer on his penis (a chancre), but he did not re-attend the clinic because it healed within a month and so he had not received any treatment.

On examination he has small irregular pupils, which accommodate, but do not react to light, and tattoos over his chest and arms. Examination of his cardiovascular system is normal. Examination of his nervous system reveals that he has lost joint position, vibration, and pain and temperature sense in his legs. Knee and ankle reflexes are absent and he is unable to stand properly with his feet together and eyes closed. His plantar responses are normal. A full blood count, vitamin B_{12} and folate levels are normal.

Questions
1 What is the likely diagnosis?
2 What investigations would you perform?
3 How would you manage this patient?

Your answers

Case 16

1 Likely diagnosis

2 Investigations

3 Management

CASE 17

see Mims 24.21

A 40-year-old acrobat goes to the sexually transmitted diseases clinic complaining of intense itching, which is especially bad at night. In addition, he is worried about some small spots that have appeared on his penis.

On examination there are a few erythematous papules and excoriated areas on the glans penis.

Questions
1 What is the probable diagnosis?
2 What investigations would help you make the diagnosis?
3 How would you manage this patient?

Notes for revision

Your answers

Case 17

1 Likely diagnosis

2 Investigations

3 Management

CASE 16

Answers

1 Likely diagnosis

Tertiary syphilis presenting with Argyll Robertson pupils (accommodation but no reaction to light) and tabes dorsalis (dorsal root column demyelination).

2 Investigations

- Non-specific tests include the VDRL (Venereal Disease Reference Laboratory test), rapid plasma reagin or cardiolipin antigen tests.
- Specific tests: treponema pallidum haemagglutination assay (TPHA) and fluorescent treponemal antibody FTA-absorbed (FTA-abs).

Serum and CSF specimens were tested using these tests. The results were:

Serum	VDRL	positive: titre 512
	TPHA	positive
	FTA-abs	positive
CSF	VDRL	positive: titre 512
	TPHA	positive
	FTA-abs	positive

3 Management

Admit him to hospital for treatment. This involves giving corticosteroids before, and then for three days after, antibiotic treatment which is intramuscular procaine penicillin. This is given for three weeks together with probenecid to reduce renal clearance of the penicillin. Corticosteroids are part of the treatment due to the occurrence of the Jarisch–Herxheimer reaction which may occur on treating individuals with active syphilis when their condition may transiently worsen shortly after starting treatment. This is thought to result from the release of treponemal antigen from 'antibiotic-assaulted' spirochaetes.

Lifestyle and health counselling should be discussed and contact tracing performed. He should be followed up regularly with further serological tests and a repeat lumbar puncture after 3–6 months. The VDRL test titre is a marker of active inflammation. It is useful in monitoring treatment response and the CSF VDRL titre should fall, as should the CSF white cell count and protein concentration.

CASE 17

Answers

1 Likely diagnosis

Scabies due to the mite *Sarcoptes scabei*. The differential diagnosis is pubic lice (*Phthirus pubis*).

2 Investigations

A diagnosis of scabies is made after suspected burrows were demonstrated by applying ink to the skin. They are caused by this parasite as it burrows into the skin where the females lay their eggs. Scrape the skin overlying the burrow to demonstrate the presence of mites or eggs on direct microscopy using a wet preparation.

3 Management

There are various choices of treatments to eradicate the mite including benzyl-benzoate, gammabenzene hexachloride, or malathion. These are applied topically over the body surface and should be left on for a period of time. The solution should be reapplied after hand washing to ensure that no transfer of mites can occur after scratching the lesions. Usually two treatments are given to ensure eradication and antihistamines may help reduce the itching.

Family members and intimate contacts should also receive treatment. Spread occurs by direct contact and via infected clothes so all clothes and bed linen shoud be dry cleaned or given a thorough hot wash.

CASE 18

see Mims 25.25–25.28

A 24-year-old astrologer with a history of intravenous drug abuse sees his doctor because he has felt tired and unwell for the last few weeks. He has noticed that his urine is very dark, he feels nauseated, and does not feel like eating, and he has developed right-sided abdominal discomfort. A friend thinks that he looks 'yellow'.

On examination he is tattooed, has yellow sclera, and is tender in the right upper quadrant of his abdomen. His liver is enlarged, firm, and smooth. The results of investigations including the liver function tests are shown in Fig. 6.1.

FIG. 6.1 RESULTS OF INVESTIGATIONS	
Investigation	**Result**
Full blood count	Normal
AST	1200 IU/l
ALT	1000 IU/l
ALP	100 IU/l
Bilirubin	60 micromol/l

Questions

1 What is the most likely diagnosis and what is the differential diagnosis of a viral hepatitis in this setting?
2 What investigations would you perform?
3 How would you manage him?
4 What other factors are important regarding control of infection?

Notes for revision

Your answers

1 Most likely diagnosis and differential diagnosis of a viral hepatitis in this setting

2 Investigations

3 Management

4 Control of infection

CASE 18

Answers

1 Most likely diagnosis and differential diagnosis of a viral hepatitis in this setting

Most likely diagnosis is acute hepatitis B infection (HBV).

Differential diagnosis includes hepatitis A, hepatitis C, delta hepatitis (as a hepatitis B coinfection/superinfection), cytomegalovirus (CMV) infection, and Epstein–Barr virus (EBV) infection.

2 Investigations

- Collect a clotted blood specimen for hepatitis B surface antigen (HBsAg) testing and markers of HBV infection (see below).
- HBsAg testing: using ELISA and the reverse passive haemagglutination (RPHA) test. The RPHA test allows an estimation of the HBsAg titre. The potential pitfall of the ELISA monoclonal antibody-based assay is that it is extremely specific and may not detect any of the rare HBV escape mutants with mutations in the region to which that monoclonal antibody has been made. The RPHA is a polyclonal-based test and should detect these mutants.
- Anti-HB core IgM.
- Anti-HB core (total IgM and IgG).
- HBeAg.

The results of these investigations are as follows: HBsAg EIA positive (confirmed by specific neutralisation with immune serum containing antibody to the HBsAg); HBsAg RPHA titre 1:1280; anti-HB core IgM positive; anti-HB core (total IgM and IgG) positive; HBeAg positive.

These results are consistent with an acute HBV infection.

- If the sample is HBsAg negative, test for HAV IgM and HCV antibody. HCV antibody would not be detected at this early stage by enzyme immunoassay (EIA) because anti-HCV seroconversion may be delayed for several months after an acute HCV infection. The test is usually repeated two months later if clinically indicated.

3 Management

- Repeat the HBV serology in one, three, and six months to see whether the infection resolves. If HBsAg is still present after six months this man is a hepatitis B carrier and should be followed up regularly because he may develop complications of chronic HBV infection (i.e. chronic active hepatitis, chronic persistent hepatitis, hepatocellular carcinoma). In addition, some individuals switch from being HBeAg positive to anti-HBe positive and some lose their HBsAg and become anti-HBs positive.
- Advise him to avoid alcohol and strenuous exercise.
- He is also at risk of other infectious diseases because of his intravenous drug abuse and this should be discussed with him in the general context of health counselling.

4 Control of infection

HBV infection is a notifiable disease in the UK. Sexual partners or individuals with whom he has shared needles should be followed up, counselled and tested to see whether they have serological evidence of a past hepatitis B infection as a matter of urgency. If there is no evidence of past HBV infection these individuals should be offered a course of hepatitis B immunisation together with an injection of hepatitis B hyperimmuneglobulin (HBIG) to attenuate/modify/prevent HBV infection.

CASE 19

see Mims 25.13–25.14

An 11-month-old baby girl is admitted to the paediatric unit with a two-day history of fever, vomiting, and copious watery diarrhoea. She was a full-term normal delivery and has two siblings, one of whom had a mild diarrhoeal illness that cleared up four days earlier.

On examination she is unwell, mildly dehydrated, and febrile with a temperature of 38°C. Her abdomen is soft and there are no other findings of note.

Questions

1 What would be your immediate management of this baby?
2 What viral causes of diarrhoea are most likely?
3 How would a viral infection be diagnosed?
4 What is the natural course of the infection?

Notes for revision

Your answers

1 Immediate management

2 Most likely viral causes of the diarrhoea

3 Diagnosis of a viral infection

4 Natural course of the infection

CASE 19

Answers

1 Immediate management
- Admit to a source isolation room in the ward.
- Collect blood for urea and electrolyte determination.
- Rehydrate orally unless she is vomiting, in which case intravenous fluids are needed.
- Send a stool sample to bacteriology and virology for analysis.

2 Most likely viral causes of the diarrhoea
Viral gastroenteritis can be divided into sporadic infantile gastroenteritis and epidemic viral gastroenteritis. The most common cause of sporadic infantile gastroenteritis is a rotavirus infection. Adenovirus infections are the second most common cause.

3 Diagnosis of a viral infection
- Electron microscopy (using phosphotungstic acid as a negative stain) is the method of choice because in this setting it is a 'catch-all' method that allows detection of a variety of viruses for which there are no generally available specific tests for detecting viral antigen or antibody to that antigen.
- There is a particle agglutination test that is specific for rotavirus infection. This is widely used, but may miss some rotavirus infections.
- In specialised laboratories enzyme-linked immunosorbent assays (ELISAs), radioimmunoassays (RIAs), or nucleic acid detection methods are available for some of the viruses associated with gastroenteritis.

72 nm diameter wheel-like particles are demonstrated by electron microscopy and rotaviral infection is diagnosed.

4 Natural course of the infection
If the child is dehydrated, fluid replacement therapy is needed. There is no specific treatment for any of the viral causes of diarrhoea, and rotaviral excretion should decrease within a week. Avoid lactose-based fluids as the loss of the distal parts of the intestinal villi due to viral infection results in a disaccharidase deficiency and therefore lactose intolerance/malabsorption.

The most important measures to prevent nosocomial infection are to place the child in source isolation and maintain high standards of hygiene, in particular thorough handwashing after contact with the child by any member of staff.

CASE 20

see Mims 25.30

A 30-year-old alcoholic has developed severe abdominal pain and is brought to the A&E department having been found collapsed in the train station. He vomits on admission and is feverish. His abdominal pain is made worse by movement and he looks very pale.

On examination he is shocked with a tachycardia of 110 beats/min and a weak, thready pulse, and a blood pressure of 90/60 mm Hg. His temperature is 38°C and examination of his abdomen reveals rebound tenderness and board-like rigidity.

Questions

1 A diagnosis of peritonitis and septicaemia secondary to a probable perforated viscus is made. Which bacteria may cause peritonitis in this situation?
2 How would you investigate him?
3 How would you manage him?
4 The results of the investigations are shown in Fig. 6.2. He is treated with intravenous ampicillin, gentamicin, and metronidazole and undergoes an emergency laparotomy. The findings include a perforated duodenal ulcer and peritonitis. How would you manage him further?

FIG. 6.2 RESULTS OF INVESTIGATIONS	
Investigation	**Result**
Chest radiograph	Gas under the diaphragms consistent with a perforation
Abdominal radiograph	Normal
Electrocardiogram	Normal
Haemoglobin	10 g/dl
White cell count	25 x 10^9/l with 90% neutrophils
Platelets	Normal
Urea, glucose, electrolytes and amylase	Normal
Blood cultures	Gram-negative rods detected after 12 hours' incubation

Notes for revision

Your answers

1 **Bacteria that cause peritonitis in this situation**

2 **Investigations**

3 **Management**

4 **Further management**

CASE 20

Answers

1 Bacteria that cause peritonitis in this situation
The peritoneal cavity is a sterile compartment. If a viscus is perforated the normal flora of the gastrointestinal tract, as in this case, would usually be responsible for the peritonitis.

2 Investigations
Investigations would include a full blood count and cross matching for blood transfusion, urea and electrolytes, glucose and amylase blood tests, chest and abdominal radiographs, an electrocardiogram, and blood cultures.

3 Management
Immediate management involves resuscitation using intravenous fluids, which should stabilise the cardiovascular system. Antibiotic treatment should be instituted to cover Gram-negative organisms, anaerobes, and faecal streptococci (enterococci) in particular. Possible choices include ampicillin, gentamicin, and metronidazole.

4 Further management
A peritoneal aspirate was collected and sent for bacteriological examination. The Gram stain showed numerous Gram-negative rods in the peritoneal fluid. *Escherichia coli* was isolated from both the blood cultures and peritoneal aspirate and was susceptible to ampicillin and gentamicin. Peak and trough gentamicin levels and monitoring of the blood urea and electrolytes were performed to avoid nephrotoxicity and ototoxicity, which may complicate treatment with an aminoglycoside. This patient made an uneventful recovery and the antibiotic treatment was stopped after ten days.

CASE 21

see Mims 25.29–25.30

A 50-year-old hotel manageress develops abdominal pain, which is diagnosed as acute cholecystitis. She is admitted to hospital for observation, and ultrasound of her gall bladder reveals a few gall stones. She recovers and is discharged and a date is fixed for an elective cholecystectomy when the infection has settled. She is readmitted a week later with a swinging fever and severe abdominal pain in the right hypochondrium.

On examination she is unwell with a temperature of 38°C and is tender over the right hypochondrium. There are no other relevant findings. The results of investigations are shown in Fig. 6.3.

FIG. 6.3 RESULTS OF INVESTIGATIONS	
Investigation	Result
Haemoglobin	13 g/dl
White cell count	12×10^9/l, mostly neutrophils
Platelets	300×10^9/l
Urea and electrolytes	Normal
Liver function tests	A slight rise in the liver enzymes
Chest radiograph	Small right-sided pleural effusion
Ultrasound of liver and gall bladder	A few gall stones and an echogenic area in the liver

Questions
1 What is the diagnosis and which bacteria are likely to be involved?
2 What investigations would you perform?
3 What would your further management be?

Your answers

Case 21

1 Diagnosis and bacteria likely to be involved

2 Investigations

3 Further management

CASE 22

see Mims 25.7

A 55-year-old Bangladeshi man is referred to the gastrointestinal open access endoscopy clinic. He has a two year history of recurrent intermittent dyspepsia and upper abdominal discomfort. Although the symptoms were initially relieved by antacids, for the last six months he has been treated with an H_2 antagonist. He has lost 15 kg in weight and his symptoms have been worsening.

Endoscopy shows antral gastritis and a duodenal ulcer. There is no evidence of malignancy.

Questions
1 What microbiological investigations would you consider?
2 How would you manage him?
3 What follow up would be appropriate?
4 What other diseases are associated with the underlying aetiology of this man's duodenal ulcer?

Your answers

Case 22

1 Microbiological investigations

2 Management

3 Follow up

4 Other diseases associated with the underlying aetiology of his duodenal ulcer

Notes for revision

CASE 21

Answers

1 Diagnosis and bacteria likely to be involved

Cholecystitis complicated by a hepatic abscess. The pleural effusion is 'sympathetic' due to the inflammation in the immediate area underlying the diaphragm. The likely causes are anaerobes, Gram-negative facultative anaerobes (e.g. *Escherichia*, *Klebsiella* sp.), and streptococci such as *Streptococcus milleri*.

2 Investigations

- Blood cultures.
- Surgical drainage/ultrasound-guided fine needle aspiration of the abscess and Gram stain of the pus that is collected.

Gram-negative rods and Gram-positive cocci in chains were detected in the pus. A drain was inserted and treatment started with ampicillin, gentamicin, and metronidazole.

3 Further management

She should have a cholecystectomy when she has recovered.

....

CASE 22

Answers

1 Microbiological investigations

- Culture of the gastric biopsy with particular conditions for the growth of *Helicobacter pylori*. A microaerophilic environment as used for the isolation of *Campylobacter* species is required. *H. pylori* is a spiral-shaped Gram-negative rod, similar in appearance to *Campylobacters*.
- Serum can be tested to look for the presence of antibodies to *H. pylori*.

H. pylori was cultured from the gastric biopsy.

2 Management

Antimicrobial therapy is necessary for patients infected with *H. pylori* to eradicate the organism. Several regimens have been reported, and the most effective are those involving a combination of antimicrobials and an H_2 antagonist, of which metronidazole is the most important component. Common regimens include metronidazole, amoxycillin, and bismuth sub-salicylate or omeprazole, metronidazole, and amoxycillin.

3 Follow up

He should be reviewed in the clinic after two months of therapy to repeat the gastric biopsy for *H. pylori*. A ^{13}C urea breath test can also be used to detect *H. pylori*. This works on the principle that if *H. pylori* is present, ^{13}C-labelled urea will be split by these urease containing organisms into $^{13}CO_2$, which can then be detected. Serology is unhelpful because it may take several months before a patient becomes seropositive.

4 Other diseases associated with the underlying aetiology of his duodenal ulcer

H. pylori infection is the major causative agent of chronic antral gastritis, and is associated with both gastric and duodenal ulceration. It has been suggested that *H. pylori* plays a key role in the development of gastric lymphoma and possibly gastric carcinoma.

Notes for revision

CASE 23

see Mims 25.2–25.10

An 18-year-old art student presents with a history of diarrhoea. He has just returned from a three-month visit to India. During the first weeks of his visit he developed diarrhoea, which settled without treatment. A few days before his return he developed more severe diarrhoea associated with abdominal pain and a loss of appetite. He is passing several small volume stools a day, which are blood stained.

On examination he is thin and dehydrated. He has generalised abdominal tenderness and active bowel sounds. Other systems are normal. The results of investigations are shown in Fig. 6.4.

FIG. 6.4 RESULTS OF INVESTIGATIONS	
Investigation	Result
Haemoglobin	14 g/dl
White cell count	12×10^9/l with 80% neutrophils
Abdominal radiograph	Normal

Questions

1 What pathogens may be responsible for this illness?
2 What further investigations are necessary to establish which pathogen is responsible?
3 What control of infection measures are necessary if he is admitted to hospital?

Notes for revision

Your answers

1 Possible pathogens

2 Further investigations

3 Control of infection measures if he is admitted to hospital

CASE 23

Answers

1 Possible pathogens

Bloody diarrhoea is usually a symptom of dysentery. The pathogens that can cause dysentery are *Shigella* species, *Escherichia coli* O157/H7 (entero-haemorrhagic *E. coli* (EHEC) or verocytotoxic *E. coli* (VTEC)), enteroinvasive *E. coli* (EIEC), and *Entamoeba histolytica*. *Campylobacter* species can also produce a bloody diarrhoea, but are not usually associated with pus.

2 Further investigations

A stool sample for the investigation of bacteria and parasites may help to establish the responsible organism. Ova and cysts of parasites can be identified in a faecal concentrate preparation. The trophozoites of *E. histolytica* can be visualised in a freshly passed faecal sample brought to the laboratory immediately. The stool sample should be cultured on to media that is selective for intestinal pathogens and suppresses the majority of normal bowel flora. *Salmonella* and *Shigella* are examples of non-lactose fermenters. *Campylobacter* species grow in a microaerophilic environment at 42°C. Where VTEC is a possible pathogen, sorbitol MacConkey agar should be used. VTEC are non-sorbitol fermenters – a differentating feature.

3 Control of infection measures if he is admitted to hospital

Care would be necessary to ensure that the infection does not spread to any other patients. He should be nursed in a side-room in source isolation. All staff should wear plastic disposable aprons during patient contact and wash their hands thoroughly on completing their task. Particular care should be exercised when dealing with bed pans containing faeces.

If he is not admitted, or on discharge back home, he should be made aware of the faeco-oral route of transmission. Advice should be given on hand washing after micturition and defaecation. If possible he should not handle food while he has diarrhoea. If he needs to prepare food, he must take care to wash his hands first.

CASE 24

see Mims 25.12

A 60-year-old African man presents with a four-day history of watery diarrhoea, abdominal pain, and distension. No one else in his family is affected, and he has not visited Africa recently. He is known to have chronic obstructive airways disease and a month ago presented with a six-day history of a worsening cough producing a greenish-coloured sputum, and dyspnoea at rest. Sputum cultures grew *H. influenzae*, sensitive to amoxycillin. He completed the prescribed course of amoxycillin three weeks ago.

On examination he is apyrexial, although he is rather dyspnoeic and restless. His pulse rate is 100 beats/min and blood pressure 120/80 mm Hg. His abdomen is diffusely tender, with some suggestion of guarding over the lower half. He was referred for a surgical opinion.

Questions
1 What is the differential diagnosis?
2 What is the mechanism of disease production?
3 How is this condition best managed?

Notes for revision

Your answers

1 **Differential diagnosis**

2 **Mechanism of disease production**

3 **Management**

CASE 24

Answers

1 Differential diagnosis

Although he is from Africa, and food poisoning organisms are frequently responsible for diarrhoea, the history of recent antibiotic treatment suggests the diagnosis of antibiotic-associated diarrhoea. This condition may cause pseudomembranous colitis, which may lead to a toxic megacolon. The organism responsible is *Clostridium difficile*. A sigmoidoscopy was performed and severe pseudomembranous colitis was confirmed.

2 Mechanism of disease production

The normal flora of the gut is important in controlling the local environment, protecting the bowel from invasion due to pathogens. The anaerobes of the gut are most important in maintaining this 'colonisation resistance'. Antibiotic consumption destroys a large part of the normal flora, allowing overgrowth of some of the components that are normally suppressed. *Cl. difficile* overgrows in these conditions and produces disease by producing two toxins, a cyclotoxin and an enterotoxin. They damage the epithelium of the gut and in the most severe cases cause pseudomembranous colitis.

The presence of the toxin can be detected in the laboratory by finding a cytotoxic effect in cell culture that is neutralised by antibody specific to the toxin. More recently, a latex agglutination test and ELISA to detect the toxin have become commercially available.

3 Management

Cl. difficile colitis is treated with oral vancomycin or metronidazole. The vancomycin is not absorbed, and remains in high concentrations in the bowel lumen. It is not necessary to measure serum levels when oral vancomycin is instituted as would apply when using intravenous vancomycin.

It is necessary to source isolate patients with pseudomembranous colitis if hospitalised because outbreaks of *Cl. difficile*-associated diarrhoea in hospitals have been well documented.

CASE 25

A 35-year-old Bangladeshi maths teacher presents to A&E having returned to the UK from Bangladesh three weeks ago. While there he was unwell with a fever and diarrhoea. This seemed to settle down, but for the last two weeks he has been feeling weak and listless and has become constipated. He also describes aching joints. He had visited his doctor who had given him a course of antibiotics, but this had not improved his symptoms.

On examination he is unwell with a fever and is mildly dehydrated. Examination reveals no lymphadenopathy and his chest is clear. There is some diffuse tenderness in his abdomen.

Questions

1 What are the major causes of a pyrexia of unknown origin (PUO) in an individual from the Indian subcontinent?
2 What investigations would you arrange?
3 How is this condition transmitted?
4 How should he be managed in hospital?

CASE 26

A two-year-old boy is referred to the paediatricians with a 24-hour history of vomiting and diarrhoea. He is very floppy and listless and the parents, one of whom is a surgeon, are most anxious. He is normally a happy playful child and is up to date with immunisations. No one else in the family is unwell and his mother is seven months pregnant.

On examination he is mildly dehydrated and his temperature is 37.5°C. Ear, nose, and throat examination is normal, and his chest is clear. His abdomen is soft, and he complains of a mild tenderness in the lower quadrants.

Questions

1 How would you investigate him?
2 The results of investigations are shown in Fig. 6.5. How would you manage this child?
3 What control of infection measures are necessary?

FIG. 6.5 RESULTS OF INVESTIGATIONS	
Investigation	**Result**
Full blood count	Normal
Urea and electrolytes	Normal
Blood cultures	Negative
Stool virology investigations	Negative
Stool microbiology	*Salmonella* sp. isolated

Notes for revision

see Mims 25.22–25.23

Your answers

Case 25

1 Major causes of PUO in an individual from the Indian subcontinent

2 Investigations

3 Mechanism of transmission

4 Management in hospital

see Mims 25.5–25.6

Your answers

Case 26

1 Investigation

2 Management

3 Control of infection measures

CASE 25

Answers

1 Major causes of a pyrexia of unknown origin (PUO) in an individual from the Indian subcontinent

Malaria, typhoid, and tuberculosis are all possible diagnoses of a PUO in an individual who comes from Bangladesh. This man's symptomatology is consistent with typhoid.

2 Investigations

Investigations should include the following:
- Full blood count.
- Urea and electrolytes.
- If tuberculosis is a possibility, a chest radiograph.
- Thick and thin blood film to exclude malaria.
- Blood cultures to diagnose typhoid.
- Urine and faecal examination and culture may reveal *Salmonella typhi*.

Gram-negative rods were identified one day after admission as *S. typhi*.

3 Mechanism of transmission

There is no animal reservoir of *S. typhi*. All patients have therefore ingested food or drink that has been contaminated by a typhoid carrier. Unlike the salmonellas that produce food poisoning, the dose required to produce infection is low.

4 Management in hospital

When he is admitted, he should be nursed in source isolation with excretion/secretion precautions. He should be rehydrated with intravenous fluids if necessary, and given an appropriate antimicrobial agent. Ciprofloxacin is being increasingly used because resistance to ampicillin, chloramphenicol, and cotrimoxazole is described in the Indian subcontinent. There is also some suggestion that it may reduce the rate of asymptomatic carriage, unlike the other antimicrobials used to treat *S. typhi*.

···

CASE 26

Answers

1 Investigation

He probably has an infective diarrhoea. However, it is important to consider a urinary tract infection. Base-line investigations should include a stool sample, which should be sent to virology and bacteriology, and urine cultures. As the child is so unwell, blood cultures, a full blood count and urea and electrolyte determination should be performed.

2 Management

He should be admitted to a side-room in source isolation with enteric precautions. It may be appropriate to give him intravenous fluids if he continues to vomit. Antidiarrhoeal and antimicrobial agents are not usually given, but if he was septicaemic, antimicrobial drugs must be given.

3 Control of infection measures

In the UK his infection must be notified to the local Department of Public Health so that possible sources of the *Salmonella* sp. infection can be investigated further.

OBSTETRIC AND PERINATAL INFECTIONS

CASE 27

see Mims 26.5–26.6

A paediatrician is called to the postnatal ward by a midwife. She is anxious about a baby boy born 12 hours ago. The child is the mother's first baby. The labour was long and the delivery difficult and eventually forceps had to be used. The mother's membranes ruptured 12 hours before the baby was born. The mother had a fever of 38.5°C during the last stages of labour, which has persisted since her arrival on the postnatal ward.

The baby had Apgar scores of 1 at 1 minute and 9 at 5 minutes. On examination the baby is lethargic and pale. He has a faint systolic murmur, crepitations in both lung fields, and his liver is palpable below the costal margin. He is transferred to the Special Care Unit.

Questions

1 What is the likely diagnosis and what are the likely pathogens?
2 How would you investigate this baby?
3 What are the risk factors in his mother's history?

Your answers

1 Likely diagnosis and likely pathogens

2 Investigation

3 Risk factors in the mother's history

Notes for revision

CASE 27

Answers

1 Likely diagnosis and likely pathogens

The baby is septicaemic. The most likely pathogens responsible for septicaemia in the newborn are organisms acquired from the mother's genital tract. Group B streptococci are the most common, but *Escherichia coli* and *Listeria monocytogenes* are also important pathogens in this age group.

2 Investigation

The baby should have a septic screen. In particular, this involves a blood culture and cerebrospinal fluid (CSF) sample. Deep ear swabs and a gastric aspirate may help to identify the pathogen responsible. A maternal vaginal swab should also be taken. Antimicrobial therapy should be started before the results of cultures are known and there are many different regimens which may be used. Common combinations are cefotaxime and benzylpenicillin, or ampicillin and gentamicin. The use of aminoglycosides requires careful monitoring of pre and post serum levels to minimise toxicity. Once the pathogen has been identified, the antibiotic regimen can be tailored accordingly.

Group B streptococci were isolated from this baby's blood culture and he was treated with intravenous benzylpenicillin and gentamicin.

3 Risk factors in the mother's history

The maternal history that points to an increased risk of neonatal infection include the following:
- Early rupture of membranes.
- Maternal pyrexia.
- A long and difficult labour.

CASE 28

A 30-year-old woman has had a caesarean section for fetal distress. One day after the operation she is noticed to be confused. The next day her confusion has increased and she has developed a temperature. Her abdominal wound is red and inflamed. She deteriorates rapidly and develops respiratory distress and is sent to the Intensive Therapy Unit (ITU).

On arrival on ITU, her pulse rate is 140 beats/min and her blood pressure is 80/60 mm Hg. It is noticed that she has a widespread bullous rash and is grossly oedematous. Her urine output is negligible. Her wound is severely inflamed and is oozing blood-stained fluid. Her fingers and toes are dusky purple. The results of initial investigations are shown in Fig. 7.1.

FIG. 7.1 RESULTS OF INVESTIGATIONS	
Investigation	Result
Haemoglobin	14 g/dl
White cell count	17.0×10^9/l with 80% neutrophils
Clotting profile	Prolonged
Urea	16 mmol/l
Creatinine	249 mmol/l

Questions

1 What is the diagnosis?
2 What are the likely pathogens and how is the disease mediated?
3 What is the appropriate antibiotic management?
4 What control of infection procedures are necessary?

Notes for revision

see Mims 28.5–28.6

Your answers

1 Diagnosis

2 Likely pathogens and how the disease is mediated

3 Appropriate antibiotic management

4 Control of infection procedures

CASE 28

Answers

1 Diagnosis

She has toxic shock syndrome (TSS). The clinical pointers are tachycardia, hypotension, confusion, swelling and bullae with late desquamation. She also has renal failure and disseminated intravascular coagulation (DIC). The morbidity and mortality (30%) of this condition is high.

2 Likely pathogens and how the disease is mediated

TSS is most frequently described in association with staphylococcal infection, but has been reported with streptococcal disease. The disease in both staphylococcal and streptococcal infection is mediated via toxin production. These toxins belong to a class of proteins known as 'superantigens'. The first reports of TSS were described in women in association with tampon use and *Staphylococcus aureus* was implicated. Since then TSS has been described after skin infection and after surgical infection, as in this case.

3 Appropriate antibiotic management

Appropriate management includes cardiovascular, respiratory, and renal support, most appropriately given in an ITU setting. Antimicrobial chemotherapy should also be given initially to cover both staphylococcal and streptococcal infection when the diagnosis of TSS is considered, until the pathogen is found.

4 Control of infection procedures

Control of infection measures are taken to prevent the spread of Group A streptococci and rarely where TSS is due to a methicillin-resistant *Staph. aureus* (MRSA). If possible, the patient should be source isolated in a side-room, to prevent aerial spread of the organism. Staff should be meticulous in their hand washing both before and after caring for the patient. Gloves and gowns should be worn when working with the patient.

Notes for revision

CASE 29

see Mims 27.8

A 20-year-old archeology student had felt unwell for a few days with a fever, headache, and sore throat. These symptoms had improved and then become much worse over the next week. He is admitted to hospital with a severe headache and photophobia.

On examination he has a fever of 38°C, neck stiffness, photophobia, and a fine erythematous rash on his trunk, face and limbs. He has no focal neurological signs. Immediately he is given intravenous benzylpenicillin, a set of blood cultures is collected, and a lumbar puncture is performed. The results of the lumbar puncture are shown in Fig. 8.1.

FIG. 8.1 RESULTS OF LUMBAR PUNCTURE	
Investigation	**Result**
CSF appearance	Clear
White cell count	200/mm^3, predominantly lymphocytic
Protein	0.4 g/l
CSF glucose	3 mmol/l
Blood glucose	4.5 mmol/l
Gram stain	No organisms were seen

Questions

1 What is the most likely diagnosis?
2 What are the common viral causes of this clinical picture in descending order of frequency and how can they be differentiated?
3 How would you manage him?

Notes for revision

Your answers

1 Most likely diagnosis

2 Common viral causes of an aseptic meningitis in descending order of frequency and how they can be differentiated

3 Management

CASE 29

Answers

1 Most likely diagnosis

Aseptic (viral) meningitis, especially as the ratio of CSF : blood glucose levels was normal and no organisms are seen on the Gram stain.

Although the history is more suggestive of a viral cause, if a patient presents with meningitis and a rash, meningococcal infection must be considered. It may be a life-saving measure to give an intravenous bolus of benzylpenicillin immediately before doing anything else, providing the patient is not allergic to penicillin, in which case an alternative antibiotic should be given (i.e. chloramphenicol).

2 Common viral causes of an aseptic meningitis in descending order of frequency and how they can be differentiated

- Enteroviral infections, including echoviruses and coxsackieviruses.
- Mumps.
- Herpes simplex types 1 and 2.

Clinically it is possible to differentiate between these viral infections: most patients with mumps will have a parotitis, whereas patients with HSV type 2 infections (and sometimes HSV type 1) may have genital herpes lesions.

3 Management

- Admit to a source isolation room.
- Notify the infection; all cases of acute meningitis should be notified in the UK.
- Send a throat swab, and stool and CSF sample for viral isolation and a serum sample for enterovirus-specific IgM determination (and mumps serology if pertinent).
- Give pain relief for the headache.

CASE 30

see Mims 27.8–27.11

A 45-year-old bank manageress is brought to hospital by ambulance having collapsed in the street. She is unable to give a history, but a passer-by had said that she suddenly collapsed having left a shop and then had a seizure. The police contact her husband who tells them that she has been complaining of a headache for the past few days and has been acting in a slightly strange way. She has no relevant past medical history, has not had a seizure before, and is on no medication.

On examination she is drowsy, confused, and has a temperature of 38°C. She has no focal neurological signs, although her reflexes are brisk. The rest of her examination is normal. Fundoscopy reveals no papilloedema and examination of the oropharynx and ears is normal.

Investigations include a full blood count, which is normal, and urea and electrolytes, including a glucose level, which are also normal.

Questions

1 What urgent investigations would you perform?
2 The result of the computerised axial tomography (CT scan) and a lumbar puncture are given in Fig. 8.2. What diagnoses would you consider in the light of these results and the clinical history?

FIG. 8.2 RESULTS OF INVESTIGATIONS	
Investigation	**Result**
CT scan	An area of low density attenuation in the left temporal lobe; no evidence of cerebral oedema or midline shift
CSF appearance	Clear
White cell count	50/mm^3, all lymphocytes
Red cells	Zero
Protein	0.9 g/dl
CSF glucose	3.3 mmol/l
Blood glucose	5 mmol/l
Gram stain	No organisms seen

3 How would you manage and treat her?

Notes for revision

Your answers

1 Urgent investigations

2 Diagnoses

3 Management and treatment

CASE 30

Answers

1 Urgent investigations

A CT scan of her head followed by a lumbar puncture if the CT scan does not demonstrate raised intracranial pressure.

2 Diagnoses

It is important to rule out a subarachnoid haemorrhage, a subdural haemorrhage (both are unlikely in the absence of red blood cells and xanthochromic appearance in the CSF), a cranial space-occupying lesion including a cerebral abscess, metabolic causes of seizures, and meningitis.

The presentation and findings are more consistent with an encephalitic process and the most common causes of a viral encephalitis include herpes simplex (HSV), mumps, and enteroviruses. More detailed clinical examination revealed the presence of genital ulcers.

3 Management and treatment

There is enough evidence to implicate HSV infection as the cause of the encephalitis and so intravenous acyclovir should be started immediately together with other general supportive measures. It is important that she is treated with acyclovir for at least two weeks to prevent a relapse. Finding diffuse slow wave activity on an electroencephalogram (EEG) would further assist in making a diagnosis. A genital swab should be collected for viral isolation and CSF should be cultured, although it is extremely unusual to isolate HSV from CSF. Finally, it is possible to detect HSV DNA in CSF specimens using the polymerase chain reaction technology (PCR) and this service may be available in some laboratories.

CASE 31

see Mims 27.7–27.8

A 24-year-old man with HIV visits his doctor with a six-week history of recurrent and worsening headaches. His CD4 count is 80 /mm^3 and he has been well since being diagnosed as HIV-1 seropositive in 1987.

On examination he has no focal neurological signs and fundoscopy is normal. He has oral candidiasis. A CT head scan is normal and a lumbar puncture is performed. The results are given in Fig. 8.3.

FIG. 8.3 RESULTS OF INVESTIGATIONS	
Investigation	**Result**
CSF appearance	Clear
White cells	150 /mm^3 predominantly lymphocytic
CSF glucose	2.2 mmol/l
Blood glucose	3.8 mmol/l
Protein	0.4 g/dl

Questions

1 What is the most likely diagnosis and what diagnostic tests would you perform?
2 What other confirmatory investigations might you ask for?
3 How would you manage him?

Notes for revision

Your answers

1 **Most likely diagnosis and diagnostic tests**

2 **Other confirmatory investigations**

3 **Management**

CASE 31

Answers

1 Most likely diagnosis and diagnostic tests

The most likely diagnosis is *Cryptococcus neoformans* (fungal) infection. The serum can be immediately tested for cryptococcal antigen and an Indian ink or nigrosin stain performed on the CSF deposit. Rapid detection of cryptococcal antigen in CSF and serum may be performed using a latex particle agglutination test.

2 Other confirmatory investigations

Culture of *C. neoformans* together with antifungal sensitivity tests, which are usually performed in reference laboratories.

Cryptococcal antigen was detected in both the serum and the CSF and capsulated yeasts were seen in the CSF.

3 Management

- Treat with antiemetics, analgesics, and intravenous amphotericin B (with or without 5 fluorocytosine) or fluconazole depending on the clinical picture.
- Continue fluconazole maintenance therapy to prevent recurrences after recovery.
- Consider that he now has two AIDS-defining diagnoses, which have prognostic implications.
- Repeat the cryptococcal antigen tests monthly for six months or if he is symptomatic. Lumbar punctures may be repeated at one and six months to monitor recovery.

CASE 32

A 5-month-old baby presents to A&E with a 12-hour history of vomiting and not feeding. She is somewhat irritable, and her mother thinks that she had a temperature, although she had not measured it. She has previously been quite well and is up to date with her immunisations.

On examination she is very flat and listless. Her temperature is 38°C and she does not have a rash. Her fontanelle is full and she cries when her head is moved. Her chest is clear and her abdomen soft, with no organomegaly.

Questions

1 What is the differential diagnosis?
2 What investigations would you perform?
3 The results of investigations are shown in Fig. 8.4. How would you manage this child and her family?

see Mims 27.3–27.5

Your answers

1 Differential diagnosis

2 Investigations

3 Management

FIG. 8.4 RESULTS OF INVESTIGATIONS	
Investigation	**Result**
Urine microscopy	<1 white blood cell/mm^3
CSF appearance	slightly turbid
White cell count	350 /mm^3, predominantly neutrophils
Red cells	10 /mm^3
Protein	1 g/l
CSF glucose	0.5 mmol/l
Blood glucose	6.4 mmol/l
Gram stain	Gram-negative diplococci
Haemoglobin	15 g/l
White cell count	22 x10^9/l with 85% neutrophils
Urea and electrolytes	Normal

4 What vaccines are currently available?

4 Current state of immunisation

Notes for revision

61

CASE 32

Answers

1 Differential diagnosis

She is septic. The differential diagnosis includes *Neisseria meningitidis*, *Haemophilus influenzae* type b, *Streptococcus pneumoniae*.

2 Investigations

She requires a septic screen, which should include the following.

- Clean catch urine.
- Blood cultures.
- CSF specimen.

Additional investigations that should be carried out are urea and electrolytes and a full blood count. These investigations show that she has meningococcal meningitis.

3 Management

She should have intravenous antibiotics. *Neisseria meningitidis* is sensitive to penicillin and high-dose intravenous benzylpenicillin should be used. Other antibiotics are used in this situation, and cefotaxime and ceftriaxone are the most common alternatives. She should also have supportive care, including intravenous fluids and nasogastric suction in the acute period.

Contacts of cases of meningococcal meningitis have a greatly increased risk of acquiring the disease (approximately 600-fold) and close household contacts should be given rifampicin for two days to eliminate the carriage of the organism from the nasopharynx. The patient should receive rifampicin after her initial treatment course, as the antibiotics used to treat meningococcal meningitis do not eradicate carriage. In the UK this is a notifiable infection.

4 Current state of immunisation

There are vaccines available, which protect against group A and C meningococci. However, they are not very effective in children under two years of age. The majority of meningococcal disease is due to group B meningococci for which there is no effective vaccine. This is an area of active research.

CASE 33

see Mims 27.6

An 80-year-old man presents with confusion, headache, and fever. He has been brought to hospital by his daughter, who visits him daily. She noticed that he was a little confused 24 hours previously, and appeared to have a cough, and thought that he might have flu. He is now much worse, and is unable to hold a conversation. He is also quite agitated. He normally lives on his own, and has been quite healthy. He smokes 20 cigarettes a day and has done so for most of his life.

On examination he is restless and confused. He does not respond appropriately to commands. He is pyrexial with a temperature of 38.5°C and tachycardic, his pulse rate being 110 beats/min. His blood pressure is 110/60 mm Hg. He has signs of consolidation in his left lower chest and is photophobic. His fundi cannot be visualised. He has neck stiffness and Kernig's sign is positive.

Questions

1 What investigations would you perform?
2 The results of investigations are given in Fig. 8.5. How would you manage him?
3 What are the complications of this condition?

Your answers

1 Investigations

2 Management

3 Complications

FIG. 8.5 RESULTS OF INVESTIGATIONS	
Investigation	**Result**
CSF appearance	turbid
White cell count	400 /mm^3 predominantly neutrophils
Red cell count	50 /mm^3
Protein	0.7 g/dl
CSF glucose	0.5 mmol/l
Blood glucose	6.3 mmol/l
Gram stain	Gram-positive diplococci
Latex agglutination test	Positive for *Streptococcus pneumoniae*
Haemoglobin	15 g/dl
White cell count	18 x 10^9/l with 90% neutrophils
Urea	35 mmol/l
Creatinine	250 mmol/l
Sodium	141 mmol/l
Potassium	5.4 mmol/l
Chest radiograph	Lobar consolidation of the left lower lobe

Notes for revision

CASE 33

Answers

1 Investigations

He has signs of both meningitis and pneumonia. Initial investigations should include a full blood count, urea and electrolytes, blood cultures, chest radiograph, and lumbar puncture. As his fundi cannot be visualised before the lumbar puncture is performed it is appropriate to perform a CT scan to detect raised intracranial pressure. Therefore blood cultures should be collected and antibiotics given before the CT scan so as not to delay treatment in this case. Postponing treatment by a few hours may lead to disastrous results.

2 Management

He has both pneumococcal meningitis and pneumonia and should be given high-dose intravenous penicillin and intravenous fluids to rehydrate him. Pneumococci with reduced susceptibility to benzylpenicillin have been reported, although rarely. Cefotaxime is usually a reliable alternative to treat the meningitis as benzylpenicillin will not reach the CSF in high enough concentrations to kill the organism.

3 Complications

Complications include mortality (particularly in the elderly), deafness, and neurological defects which will affect motor function.

CASE 34

see Mims 27.13

A 70-year-old man presents to the outpatient clinic with a three-week history of general malaise. More specifically over the last week he has noticed a throbbing headache and has lost his appetite. He feels that the left side of his body is weak and he has no energy. He has vomited on two occasions. He had an appendicectomy as a child, and smokes ten cigarettes a day. His past medical history is unremarkable. He lives on his own at home and usually manages to cope very well.

On examination, he has a temperature of 37.8°C and a pulse rate of 90 beats/min, and his blood pressure is 140/90 mm Hg. He is generally weak, more on the left than on the right and has brisk reflexes on his left-hand side. He is otherwise alert and orientated, and his vision is normal. There are no abnormal physical signs in his chest or abdomen.

Questions

1 What is the differential diagnosis and what is the most critical investigation?
2 What are the underlying predisposing causes of this condition?
3 How is he best managed?

Notes for revision

Your answers

1 **Differential diagnosis and most critical investigation**

2 **Underlying predisposing causes**

3 **Management**

CASE 34

Answers

1 Differential diagnosis and most critical investigation

He has a cranial space-occupying lesion. The most likely cause is a brain abscess, given his symptoms and a temperature. A CT scan should be performed in order to make the diagnosis. Blood cultures, a full blood count, urea, electrolytes and glucose should be collected.

2 Underlying predisposing causes

Brain abscesses can occur secondarily to a number of conditions:

- Contiguous spread from either otitis media or sinusitis: 40% of patients with brain abscesses in one survey had otitis media.
- Haematogenous spread of organisms causing bacteraemia or septicaemia, for example as a result of endocarditis .
- Trauma (which includes operative procedures), particularly if there has been a fracture in the base of the skull, but penetrating trauma can precipitate an infection.

3 Management

Brain abscesses usually require neurosurgical drainage. In addition, antibiotics should be given to cover possible pathogens such as anaerobes, and antibiotic combinations should include metronidazole. Other pathogens include *Streptococcus milleri* group and *Staphylococcus aureus*. Antibiotics which cross the blood–brain barrier and penetrate the abscess (e.g. chloramphenicol) are useful. Care should be taken to monitor the white cell count as chloramphenicol can induce neutropenia.

Notes for revision

CASE 35

A 65-year-old man in a coma is brought into A&E by ambulance. No relatives are with him and there is no history. The ambulance man says they were called by a neighbour who had seen no sign of him for two days. He lives on his own and apparently there are no known relatives.

On examination he is pyrexial with a temperature of 38.5°C. His pulse rate is 100 beats/min and his blood pressure 110/70 mm Hg. He does not respond to verbal commands and withdraws his legs in response to pain. He has marked neck stiffness. His reflexes are brisk and equal, his abdomen is soft, and his chest is clear.

Questions

1 What are the possible causes of his illness?
2 What investigations would you perform?
3 The results of the initial investigations are given in Table 8.6. How would you manage this man?

FIG. 8.6 RESULTS OF INVESTIGATIONS	
Investigation	**Result**
CT scan	No space-occupying lesion or evidence of raised intracranial pressure. It was therefore decided to proceed to lumbar puncture:
CSF appearance	slightly turbid
White cells	1160 /mm^3, predominantly neutrophils
Red cells	44 /mm^3
Protein	3.8 g/l
CSF glucose	3.7 mmol/l
Blood glucose	8.4 mmol/l
Gram stain	Scanty Gram-positive rods. The next day the laboratory reported *Listeria monocytogenes* in the CSF culture
Haemoglobin	17 g/dl
White cell count	25 x 10^9/l with 70% neutrophils
Urea	20 mmol/l
Sodium	145 mmol/l
Potassium	4.5 mmol/l

4 What other infections does this organism cause?

Notes for revision

see Mims 27.3–27.6

Your answers

1 **Possible causes**

2 **Investigations**

3 **Management**

4 **Other infections caused by this organism**

CASE 35

Answers

1 Possible causes

He could have a number of conditions, both infective and non-infective (e.g. subarachnoid haemorrhage or subdural haematoma). The most important bacterial infections to consider are as follows:

- Bacterial meningitis: most likely organisms are *Streptococcus pneumoniae*, *Listeria monocytogenes*, and *Mycobacterium tuberculosis*.
- Cerebral abscess.
- Subdural empyema.

2 Investigations

An urgent CT scan of the head is indicated. Base-line investigations should include a full blood count, urea and electrolytes, and blood cultures. If there is any delay in organising the CT scan, antibiotics should be given after taking blood cultures.

3 Management

While awaiting the results of the lumbar puncture, a bolus dose of ampicillin and chloramphenicol was given. He was admitted to the intensive therapy unit (ITU). Once the CSF Gram stain result was known the antimicrobials were changed to ampicillin and gentamicin. In spite of all the supportive care provided on the ITU, he died two days later.

4 Other infections caused by this organism

Listeria monocytogenes can also cause a febrile illness in pregnancy. This may be transmitted to the fetus and cause premature labour, severe neonatal infection, and death. Neonates may acquire the organism prenatally, and again this results in a severe infection. There is also evidence of cross-infection of *L. monocytogenes* in neonatal units. Infected babies should be isolated if possible. Staff should be made aware of the risks of transmission and take extra care with cross-infection procedures.

9 INFECTIONS OF THE SKIN, MUSCLE, JOINTS, BONES, AND HAEMOPOIETIC SYSTEM

CASE 36

A 17-year-old long distance runner is admitted to hospital with a fever, malaise, shortness of breath, and dull chest pain, which is not associated with exertion. He has been training for a marathon and over the previous couple of weeks has had an upper respiratory tract infection. There is no relevant past medical history or family history of illnesses.

On examination his temperature is 38°C and he is in great discomfort. He has a sinus tachycardia of 110 beats/min and a gallop rhythm is noted on chest auscultation. The rest of the physical examination is normal.

Questions
1 What immediate investigations would you perform?
2 What is the most likely diagnosis?
3 What specimens would you request?
4 How would you manage this man and what is his prognosis?

see Mims 28.25

Your answers

1 **Immediate investigations**

2 **Most likely diagnosis**

3 **Specimens**

4 **Management and prognosis**

Notes for revision

CASE 36

Answers

1 Immediate investigations
- Electrocardiogram.
- Chest radiograph.
- Full blood count.
- Urea and electrolytes.
- Myocardial enzymes.

The results of these investigations are shown in Fig 9.1.

FIG. 9.1 RESULTS OF INVESTIGATIONS	
Investigation	**Result**
Electrocardiogram	Non-specific ST segment and T wave abnormalities
Chest radiograph	Marginal cardiomegaly
Haemoglobin	14 g/dl
White cell count	$1 \times 10^9/l$
Urea and electrolytes	Normal
Myocardial enzymes	Normal

2 Most likely diagnosis

A viral myocarditis, which is classically associated with the enteroviruses which include coxsackie A and B and echoviruses. Other viruses associated with viral myocarditis include influenza A and B, measles, mumps, rubella, polio, adenoviruses, rabies, and members of the herpesvirus and arbovirus groups.

3 Specimens
- A throat swab and stool sample for enteroviral isolation.
- A serum sample for detection of enterovirus-specific IgM.
- If he is severely ill, it may be necessary to perform a myocardial biopsy in which case a specimen should be sent for enteroviral RNA extraction. This should be followed by *in situ* hybridisation and DNA amplification by polymerase chain reaction (PCR) in order to detect enteroviral nucleic acid.

4 Management and prognosis

Management is bed rest and continuous cardiac monitoring in a coronary care or intensive care unit, pain relief, and treatment of complications, which may include arrhythmias and cardiac failure. The use of corticosteroids is controversial.

Most patients recover fully, but a small percentage of cases are fatal if there is a severe myopericarditis. Recurrences can occur, especially a recurrent relapsing pericarditis, and cardiomyopathy may be a sequel.

Notes for revision

CASE 37

see Mims 28.22–28.24

A 22-year-old pregnant woman is admitted to the maternity ward in her 39th week of pregnancy and the following day has an uneventful delivery. Just before the delivery she notices areas of erythema and spots appearing on her face, chest, abdomen, and limbs. They become vesicular and the obstetrician contacts the virologist with a clinical diagnosis of chickenpox.

Questions

1 What investigations would you do?
2 How would you manage this woman and her baby?
3 How does acyclovir act?

Notes for revision

Your answers

Case 37

1 Investigations

2 Management
  ● Mother

  ● Baby

  ● Staff, patients, and other contacts

  ● Contacts who are pregnant and VZV IgG negative

3 Action of acyclovir

CASE 38

see Mims 28.6–28.7

A 14-year-old boy presents to A&E with a three day history of swelling and redness around an insect bite on his leg. He is also feeling a little off colour, with a fever and aches in his joints.

On examination he is slightly pyrexial and his cheeks are flushed. His right calf is swollen and tender. There is no discrete pus, but there is a break in the skin where the insect bite has been scratched, and a red line can be seen tracking up his leg. The inguinal lymph nodes in his groin are tender.

Questions

1 What is the diagnosis and what is the likely organism?
2 Which antibiotics can be used to treat this condition?

Notes for revision

Your answers

Case 38

1 Diagnosis and likely organism

2 Antibiotics for treatment

CASE 37

Answers

1 Investigations

Arrange for the woman and her baby to be moved to a side-room in source isolation. Examine her and collect vesicle fluid for varicella zoster virus (VZV) detection using electron microscopy (EM) and cell culture isolation. Herpesvirus particles are seen by EM and within nine days a typical varicella zoster virus (VZV) cytopathic effect is seen on cell culture.

2 Management

There are three considerations in this setting: the mother, her baby, and the staff and other patients, regarding the control of an infection that usually results in at least 90% transmission to susceptible individuals.

- A **mother** who is immunosuppressed due to her pregnancy, can have a complicated clinical course when infected with VZV. She may develop a pneumonitis, especially if she is a cigarette smoker. Careful monitoring of her respiratory rate and pulse rate together with a chest radiograph are important. Treatment with acyclovir, which reduces both viral shedding and increases time to lesion healing is recommended. The higher dose of acyclovir should be used as VZV is not as sensitive to this antiviral drug as herpes simplex virus.
- As the **baby** was born at the time the spots appeared no passive transfer of protective maternal VZV antibody would have occurred across the placenta. It is important to protect the baby with another form of passively administered high titre VZV-specific antibody and after consultation with the virologist, the baby should be given Zoster Immune Globulin (ZIG) as an intramuscular injection.
- **Staff, patients, and other contacts** should be asked if they have had chickenpox. Most people with a past history of chickenpox will have antibodies to VZV and should be protected. This method is not infallible and about 1 in 1000 individuals with a positive history do not have VZV-specific antibodies if they are tested serologically. If there is any doubt, serum should be tested for VZV IgG. The mother would have been infectious for two days before the appearance of the spots and so it is important to find all her contacts during that time. VZV antibody negative staff contacts may be incubating chickenpox and should not be in contact with at-risk patients from the tenth day after contact up to day 21.
- **Contacts who are pregnant and VZV IgG negative** should be offered ZIG, ideally within 72 hours of contact, though it can be administered within ten days of contact. This may prevent, but more often attenuates or modifies the infection.

3 Action of acyclovir

Acyclovir is an acyclic nucleoside analogue of guanosine and is an example of a prodrug because it has to be phosphorylated in order to be active. This reaction is performed by both host- and virally-encoded kinases. The result is that acyclovir triphosphate is formed and inhibits the viral DNA polymerase (to a much greater degree than host cell DNA polymerases) and affects the production of the viral DNA chain leading to premature DNA chain termination.

....

CASE 38

Answers

1 Diagnosis and likely organism

This is cellulitis, and it is usually caused by Group A streptococci.

2 Antibiotics for treatment

Group A streptococci are susceptible to penicillin. In a situation like this, oral amoxycillin will usually treat the condition. Erythromycin can be used for patients who are penicillin allergic.

CASE 39

A two-year-old girl develops a fine erythematous rash together with the sudden onset of a high fever. She is up to date with her immunisation schedule and her doctor sees her at home.

On examination she is unwell with a fever and rash. There are no other findings of note.

Questions

1 What is the differential diagnosis?
2 The diagnosis is invariably a clinical diagnosis, but if this child is admitted to hospital she may be further investigated. What investigations would you perform if she is admitted?

see Mims 28.24, 29.9

Your answers

Case 39

1 Differential diagnosis?

2 Investigations

CASE 40

A 26-year-old pregnant woman goes to see her doctor having developed a fine erythematous rash on her face, trunk, arms, and legs the previous day. This is her second pregnancy, which has so far been uneventful and she is now at 16 weeks' gestation. Naturally she is extremely anxious and is worried about her baby. She has been on no medication, no one else in the family had been unwell recently, and she remembers having had chickenpox and measles when she was younger. Her previous antenatal clinic booking blood sample have been tested for rubella antibodies, which have been detected. On examination there are no other findings of note.

Questions

1 What is the differential diagnosis with respect to possible viral infections?
2 How would you investigate her?
3 How would you manage her?

Notes for revision

see Mims 28.24

Your answers

Case 40

1 Differential diagnosis

2 Investigations

3 Management

CASE 39

Answers

1 Differential diagnosis?
- Roseola infantum (also called exanthema subitum) due to human herpes virus 6 (HHV 6).
- Enteroviral infections (i.e. due to echoviruses, coxsackieviruses).
- Fifth's disease due to parvovirus B19, which is unlikely because the classical presentation is red, slapped cheeks together with a fine rash.
- Measles and rubella, which are unlikely because of the clinical findings and she is up to date with her immunisation schedule.

2 Investigations
- Collect a throat swab and stool specimen for viral isolation, in particular for the enteroviruses.
- Collect a serum specimen for the following tests: HHV 6 IgM (reference laboratory test), parvovirus B19 IgM, measles-specific IgM, rubella-specific IgM, and enterovirus specific IgM.

Her fever subsided over three days and HHV 6 specific IgM was detected in the serum specimen.

....

CASE 40

Answers

1 Differential diagnosis
- Rubella.
- Parvovirus B19.
- Enteroviral infections.

2 Investigations
- Check the rubella serology result of her antenatal clinic blood sample.
- Collect a blood sample for rubella IgM, parvovirus B19 IgM, and enterovirus-specific IgM detection.
- Collect a throat swab and stool sample for viral isolation with respect to enteroviral infections.

Although rubella antibody had been detected in this woman's previous blood sample there have been reports of rubella reinfection that may lead to a congenital infection, especially if the mother has had a viraemia.

The results of investigations are given in Fig. 9.2.

FIG. 9.2 RESULTS OF INVESTIGATIONS	
Investigation	**Result**
Rubella-specific IgM	Not detected
Parvovirus B19-specific IgM	Not detected
Enterovirus-specific IgM	Detected.
Tissue cell culture from throat swab and stool samples	Enteroviruses isolated
Neutralisation test using the panel of enteroviral antisera	Echovirus type 11 was detected

3 Management

Reassure her that she has had an infection with a virus that is unlikely to affect fetal development at this stage of pregnancy.

CASE 41

see Mims 28.27–28.28

A four-year-old boy is referred to the clinic with a history of a painful arm. He fell while on a climbing frame five days ago, and lacerated his right forearm. He has become more unwell in the last 24 hours with a fever, vomiting, and abdominal pain.

On examination he is miserable, dehydrated, and feverish. His right forearm is exquisitely tender over the area of the wound. His abdomen is tender, but there is no rebound or guarding. His chest is clear.

Questions

1 What is the likely diagnosis?
2 What investigations would you perform?
3 The results of investigations are given in Fig. 9.3. How would you treat this condition?

FIG. 9.3 RESULTS OF INVESTIGATIONS	
Investigation	**Result**
Haemoglobin	15 g/dl
White cell count	24×10^9/l with 90% neutrophils
Radiograph of forearm	Soft tissue swelling over the affected area of the forearm
Blood cultures	*Staphylococcus aureus*, sensitive to flucloxacillin

Your answers

Case 41

1 Likely diagnosis

2 Investigations

3 Treatment

CASE 42

see Mims 28.28

A 75-year-old diabetic is referred to the surgical clinic with a gangrenous foot. It has been black for some time, but he fears amputation and has not visited his doctor. He has been diabetic for some years, and is controlled on oral hypoglycaemic drugs. He has had numerous admissions to hospital with ulcers on his foot. On examination his foot is dusky purple. He has no peripheral foot pulses in either leg. After a long discussion, he agrees to undergo amputation.

Two days after an above-knee amputation he is confused and disorientated. His stump is inflamed and discharging thin watery fluid, and smells foul. There is crepitus in the skin surrounding the wound. His diabetes is difficult to control.

Questions

1 What is the most likely diagnosis?
2 What investigations should be performed?
3 What treatment is necessary?
4 How can such disease be prevented?

Notes for revision

Your answers

Case 42

1 Most likely diagnosis

2 Investigations

3 Treatment

4 Prevention

CASE 41

Answers

1 Likely diagnosis

The most likely diagnosis is an acute osteomyelitis. In children of this age, it may be accompanied with a history of minor trauma. It can be difficult to diagnose, particularly if vomiting is a major part of the illness.

2 Investigations

Investigations that should be performed are as follows:
- Full blood count.
- Blood cultures.
- Radiographs of the affected area.

In acute osteomyelitis, radiographic changes usually lag behind the clinical picture. The most common pathogen in such cases is *Staphylococcus aureus.*

3 Treatment

Treatment should be commenced using intravenous flucloxacillin and oral fusidic acid while the results of cultures are awaited. Intravenous fluids and nasogastric aspiration should also be started. The limb should be immobilised by splinting, and traction will reduce the pain. Pain relief and antipyretics should also be given as appropriate.

If the patient's temperature does not settle, it may be necessary to drain any collection of pus operatively. Any pus should be sent to microbiology for culture.

....

CASE 42

Answers

1 Most likely diagnosis

The presence of crepitus in the tissue surrounding an amputation wound that is infected is highly suggestive of gas gangrene. It is caused by *Clostridium perfringens,* which is part of the normal flora of the gut and commonly colonises the skin of the thigh.

2 Investigations
- A radiograph of the area will show the extent of gas in the tissues.
- A wound swab will reveal the presence of the organism.

3 Treatment

Both medical and surgical therapy is needed. It is imperative that the wound is fully debrided, often to the fascial level, the infected tissue is removed and the wound laid open. Antibiotics should be started promptly with high-dose benzylpenicillin. It may be necessary to increase the spectrum of antimicrobial cover initially, and add metronidazole and gentamicin. Gentamicin should be used with extreme caution in this age group and serum levels should be monitored.

4 Prevention

The risks of post-operative gangrene are reduced by giving prophylactic pre-operative antibiotics. A combination of benzylpenicillin and metronidazole is suitable for such purposes, and should be used in amputations and hip replacements in particular. In contrast to most surgical prophylaxis, antibiotics should be continued for 3–5 days after surgery to prevent gas gangrene.

CASE 43

see Mims 28.26

A 35-year-old man sees his doctor with a two-day history of a painful swollen left knee joint. He is a regular rugby player and thinks that he may have twisted his leg whilst playing the previous weekend. He also reported a slight feeling of 'flu' with some generalised aching and a fever. He is normally healthy.

On examination he is flushed and his temperature is 37.8°C. His left knee is red and tender to touch. There is some swelling in the soft tissues. Movements in all directions are limited by pain. There are no palpable lymph nodes. The rest of the examination is normal.

Questions

1 What are the most common infectious causes of an acute monoarthritis?
2 What other points may be helpful in the history?
3 How is the diagnosis made?
4 What would you advise on treatment?

Notes for revision

Your answers

1 Most common infectious causes of an acute mono-arthritis

2 Other points that may be helpful in the history

3 Diagnosis

4 Treatment

CASE 43

Answers

1 Most common infectious causes of an acute monoartritis

Single joints can become infected as a result of a direct penetrating injury, or as a result of haematogenous spread. The large joints are usually affected by haematogenous spread, especially the knee and hip. Disseminated *Neisseria gonorrhoeae* infection is renowned for its ability to produce a monoarthropathy. Other organisms can spread to joints, most common is *Staphylococcus aureus* (60%), but other organisms such as non group A beta haemolytic streptococci (15%) and *Streptococcus pneumoniae* (3%) may be implicated.

2 Other points that may be helpful in the history

In an arthritis due to *N. gonorrhoeae*, there is usually a history of urethral discharge in a man. Where other organisms are involved, there is usually a source of the infecting organism, eg an infected skin wound. These points should be sought in the history.

3 Diagnosis

The most effective way of diagnosing an infected joint is to take a sample of joint fluid for analysis. In the presence of infection, there will be numerous polymorphonuclear white cells. In this case, microscopic examination of the knee fluid revealed more than 2000 white cells indicative of an inflammatory process within the joint. There may be organisms seen on the Gram stain which will give an initial guide to therapy. Culture of the fluid, including suitable media for the isolation of gonococci will demonstrate the pathogen.

4 Treatment

Treatment should involve antimicrobials to eradicate the infecting organism. Gonococci involved in joint infections are usually sensitive to penicillin although penicillin resistant strains are being increasingly reported. Ceftriaxone is being used to treat gonococcal infections in many parts of the USA.

Staphylococcal infection should be treated with flucloxacillin, depending on the antibiotic sensitivity pattern, in combination with another agent such as oral fusidic acid.

10

WORLDWIDE VIRUS INFECTIONS

CASE 44

see Mims 29.6–29.9

A 19-year-old philosophy student sees the college doctor because she has been feeling tired since starting her third term three weeks previously. She has felt feverish and sweaty, and has had a sore throat and some abdominal discomfort.

On examination she has a temperature of 38.5°C, cervical lymphadenopathy, a few palatal petechiae, an inflamed pharynx, and tender, smooth splenomegaly. The results of investigations are given in Fig. 10.1.

FIG. 10.1 RESULTS OF INVESTIGATIONS

Investigation	Result
Haemoglobin	14 g/dl
White cell count	4×10^9/l with atypical lymphocytes
ALT	300 IU/l
AST	350 IU/l

Questions

1 What is the differential diagnosis?
2 How would you investigate this woman for EBV infection?
3 The results of the monospot test are given in Fig. 10.2. How would you interpret these results?

FIG. 10.2 RESULTS OF INVESTIGATIONS

Investigation	Result
Unadsorbed serum to which the indicator horse red blood cells are added	Agglutination
GPK cells to which horse red blood cells are added	Agglutination
OCS cells to which horse red blood cells are added	No agglutination
VCA IgM and EA IgM	Positive
EA-IgG	Positive – titre 640

4 What are the more common complications of EBV infections?
5 What would be your advice to this patient?

Notes for revision

Your answers

1 **Differential diagnosis?**

2 **Investigation for EBV infection?**

3 **Interpretation of the results**

4 **Common complications**

5 **Advice**

CASE 44

Answers

1 Differential diagnosis

Epstein–Barr virus (EBV) infection (also known as infectious mononucleosis or glandular fever) or cytomegalovirus (CMV) infection.

2 Investigation for EBV infection

Paul Bunnell test or monospot for heterophile antibody. The heterophile antibody is an IgM antibody that reacts with an antigen unrelated to the host that produced the antibody. The test entails using guinea pig kidney (GPK) cells to adsorb out Forsmann antibodies, which can cause a false positive test result and ox cell stroma (OCS) cells, which adsorb out the heterophile antibody.

The serum specimen is pipetted in three places onto a test card.

- Nothing is added to the first (unadsorbed) serum.
- GPK cells are added to the second serum.
- OCS cells are added to the third.

Finally the indicator horse red blood cells are added to all three specimens and the cards are gently shaken. Agglutination should occur in only two of the three tests, as the OCS cells absorb the heterophile antibody and no agglutination occurs.

In order to confirm the result the specimen should be tested for Viral Capsid Antigen (VCA)-IgM and IgG and Early Antigen (EA)-IgG.

The positive VCA-IgM and high titre EA-IgG indicate an acute EBV infection.

3 Interpretation of the results

These results are consistent with the presence of heterophile antibody and an acute EBV infection.

4 Common complications

- Hepatitis and hepatomegaly in 15–20%.
- Splenomegaly in up to 50–60%.
- Jaundice in 5–10%.
- Secondary bacterial infections (i.e. beta haemolytic streptococci) in 25%.
- Occasionally neurological and haematological complications.

5 Advice

- Rest.
- Avoid contact sports until symptoms improve.
- No alcohol until hepatitis resolves.

11

VECTOR-BORNE INFECTIONS

CASE 45

see Mims 30.8

A 42-year-old businessman is admitted to hospital with a fever, sore throat, chills, headache, muscle aches, abdominal pain, nausea and vomiting. He has returned from a 3-month trip to Sierra Leone two weeks ago and has taken antimalarial prophylaxis.

On examination he has a fever of 38°C, a mildly inflamed pharynx, a regular pulse rate of 100 beats per minute and a blood pressure of 110/70 mm Hg. The only other features of note are of splenomegaly and a tender, mildly enlarged liver.

Questions

1 What differential diagnosis must you consider immediately?
2 What immediate investigations would you perform?
3 How would you manage this patient?

Your answers

1 Diagnosis

2 Immediate investigations

3 Management

Notes for revision

CASE 45

Answers

1 Differential diagnosis

Malaria, viral haemorrhagic fever and typhoid fever.

If someone has a history of travel to such an area and develops this clinical picture within three weeks of their return, then the risk of having a viral haemorrhagic fever must be considered. This is important as these patients are placed in a category of suspicion of illness risk which is graded as minimal, moderate or strong. The type of hospital isolation unit to which the patient is admitted depends on this risk assessment. This patient was graded as a medium risk and was admitted to a high security unit in which he could be investigated and treated. In addition, any individuals in close contact with him should be contacted as they may be at risk.

2 Immediate investigations

After the patient is transferred to the high security isolation unit which contains its own laboratory, a full blood count including a differential cell count and thick and thin films, blood urea, electrolytes and glucose, an electrocardiogram, a midstream urine (MSU) specimen and stool and blood cultures should be collected.

A picture of a haemolytic anaemia, leucopaenia and a slightly lowered platelet count was seen in this case. The thin film revealed normal size, multiple infected red blood cells and approximately 10% of the red blood cells contained flimsy ring forms (malarial trophozoites). A diagnosis of falciparum malaria was made.

A serum sample should be sent for arboviral serology as individuals from endemic areas could present with dual infections.

3 Management

Full supportive care and treatment with intravenous quinine. Monitoring of haematological and biochemical parameters should be instituted, in particular measuring the level of parasitaemia in response to treatment, blood glucose and renal function.

This patient made an uneventful recovery and was found to have had chloroquine resistant falciparum malaria.

12 MULTISYSTEM ZOONOSES

CASE 46

see Mims 31.9–31.10

A 39-year-old sailor who has just finished a three-month commission in the Far East and then Africa visits his doctor having felt unwell for the previous month with a fever, headaches, tiredness, and sweats. While at sea he had recorded his temperature as 38°C . He has no other symptoms of note.

On examination he has a temperature of 39°C. The only other finding is tenderness in the left upper quadrant of his abdomen and one fingerbreadth splenomegaly. His doctor arranges for him to be admitted to hospital where he is investigated. The results of investigations are given in Fig. 12.1.

FIG. 12.1 RESULTS OF INVESTIGATIONS	
Investigation	**Result**
Haemoglobin	14 g/dl
White cell count	1.8×10^9/l
Platelets	250×10^9/l
Thick and thin blood film	No malarial parasites seen
Erythrocyte sedimentation rate (ESR)	40 mm/hr
Urea and electrolytes	Normal
Liver function tests	Normal
Chest radiograph	Normal
Blood cultures	No growth after 48 hours
Early morning urine	No growth of *Mycobacterium tuberculosis*

Questions

1 He has a pyrexia of unknown origin (PUO) and there is a wide differential diagnosis. What further questions would you ask to help make the diagnosis?
2 He had a fever, sweats, malaise and splenomegaly together with a leucopenia, what is the most likely diagnosis?
3 How would you investigate him further?
4 How would you manage him?

Notes for revision

Your answers

1 Questions asked to help make the diagnosis

2 Most likely diagnosis

3 Further investigation

4 Management

CASE 46

Answers

1 Questions to ask to help make the diagnosis

Asking about an individual's occupation is always important. This man is a sailor who has travelled to the Far East as well as Africa. Questions should be asked about:

- His lifestyle.
- Contact with any cases of infectious disease, pets or animals.
- Whether he has been bitten by any insects.
- Whether he has had any unpasteurised milk/cream or eaten any goats' cheese.

These questions may be critical in determining the cause of a PUO. In fact, he had drunk some milk in Africa directly after milking a few cows.

2 Most likely diagnosis

Brucellosis is the most likely diagnosis.

3 Further investigation

- Collect blood cultures and use a special biphasic (solid/liquid) medium called Casteñadas medium which should be incubated in CO_2 for up to six weeks.
- Test serum using the standard tube agglutination test for *Brucella* agglutinins and *Brucella* complement fixation test (CFT). A single serum tested by CFT had a titre of 2048.

4 Management

Treatment with doxycycline and rifampicin for six weeks, but relapses occur.

CASE 47

see Mims 31.8

An 18-year-old canoeist is admitted as an emergency having had a flu-like illness followed by a fever and jaundice. His parents have also noticed that he is not paying much attention to everyday matters and has become less alert. He has no relevant past medical history.

On examination he is easily distractable and has a subconjunctival haemorrhage, jaundice, and marginal hepatomegaly. The results of investigations are given in Fig. 12.2.

FIG. 12.2 RESULTS OF INVESTIGATIONS	
Investigation	**Result**
Haemoglobin	14 g/dl
White cell count	5×10^9/l
Platelets	250×10^9/l
Urea	25 mmol/l
Creatinine	190 micromol/l
Sodium	120 mmol/l
Potassium	4.9 mmol/l
Bilirubin	15 micromol/l
ALP	300 IU/l
AST	90 IU/l
ALT	70 IU/l
Urinalysis	Proteinuria and haematuria

Questions

1 What is the most likely diagnosis?
2 What investigations would you perform to make the diagnosis?
3 How would you manage this patient?
4 How did he contract this disease and what occupations are associated with this infection? What preventive measures could be instituted to avoid infection?

Your answers

1 Most likely diagnosis

2 Investigations

3 Management

4 Preventive measures

Notes for revision

CASE 47

Answers

1 **Most likely diagnosis**

The most likely diagnosis is leptospirosis. An atypical pneumonia, for example *Legionella pneumophila* infection, and viral hepatitis form part of the differential diagnosis.

2 **Investigations**
- An alkalinised urine sample should be examined by dark ground microscopy for leptospira.
- Leptospira may be isolated in special blood culture media collected in the first week of illness. This is often performed in reference laboratories.
- Serum samples can be tested for the presence of leptospiral antibodies using complement fixation tests and microagglutination tests.

3 **Management**

Treatment with intravenous benzylpenicillin and careful observation of renal function in particular. Severe cases may need monitoring in an intensive care setting.

4 **Preventive measures**

Rats' urine infected with *Leptospira icterohaemorrhagiae* may contaminate recreational and other waters. People who take part in water sports such as canoeing, sewer and abbatoir workers, and individuals who work in rodent control are at risk of infection. Protective clothing is therefore an extremely important measure, especially covering mucous membranes and cuts or abrasions.

CASE 48

see Mims 32.5–32.8

A 60-year-old woman presents to the clinic with a seven-day history of malaise, nausea, and loss of appetite. Ten years ago she was admitted with an aortic root dissection. This was corrected successfully at operation and her aortic root and valve were replaced. She has been quite well until now, although she is a poor complier and it has been difficult to stabilise her anticoagulant therapy.

On examination her temperature is 38°C. She is flushed and unwell. Her pulse rate is 110 beats/min, and her blood pressure is 80/60 mmHg. A prosthetic valvular click and a systolic murmur are heard on auscultation. Her chest is otherwise clear and abdominal examination is unremarkable. The results of initial investigations are given in Fig. 13.1.

FIG. 13.1 RESULTS OF INVESTIGATIONS	
Investigation	Result
Haemoglobin	8.3 g/dl normochromic, normocytic film
White cell count	14.6×10^9/l with 60% neutrophils
Platelets	192×10^9/l

Questions

1 What is the probable diagnosis and what further investigations are critical?
2 What is the most common pathogen responsible for this condition?
3 What are the crucial components of management of this condition?
4 What are the possible complications of this condition?
5 What guidelines are available to reduce the risk of this disease occurring?

Notes for revision

Your answers

1 Probable diagnosis and critical further investigations

2 Most common pathogen

3 Crucial components of management

4 Possible complications

5 Guidelines to reduce the risk of this disease occurring

CASE 48

Answers

1 Probable diagnosis and critical further investigations

It is probable that she has infectious endocarditis. She has an artificial aortic valve which makes this diagnosis highly likely given the presence of a fever and a murmur. In these circumstances it is important to take blood cultures to identify the pathogen responsible. At least three sets of cultures should be taken on three separate occasions to ensure the highest chances of isolating the organism. An echocardiogram, which is most sensitive if performed by a transoesophageal approach should be performed. The presence of vegetations on echocardiography are diagnostic, although their absence does not exclude the diagnosis.

2 Most common pathogen

Streptococci, usually of the viridans type, found as part of the normal flora of the mouth are the most common organisms responsible in endocarditis. However, with the increasing use of cardiac surgery to replace damaged valves, staphylococci, both *Staphylococcus aureus* and coagulase-negative staphylococci (CNS) are important. CNS are especially implicated in prosthetic valvular endocarditis. Many other organisms have been implicated as the cause of endocarditis, including some fastidious Gram-negative rods, and more unusually, fungi.

The majority of cases of endocarditis used to be due to rheumatic valve disease as a consequence of rheumatic fever. An increasing number of cases are associated with prosthetic valves, and staphylococci are the most prominent organisms found in this group of patients. Infection can be acquired at the time of surgery, when it will present within the first few months postoperatively, and usually is manifest within a few weeks. Alternatively it may present later, as in this case, when it is the result of organisms settling on the valve during a bacteraemia. The classical signs of endocarditis may not be present in this group and the patient may present more acutely.

Her blood cultures revealed *Staphylococcus aureus* in all three sets.

3 Crucial components of management

It is essential that a physician, a surgeon, and a microbiologist are involved at an early stage. It may be necessary to remove an infected valve surgically if there is no response to antimicrobial therapy. A multidisciplinary team is best placed to make such a decision for each individual case.

4 Possible complications

The most serious complications include abscess formation within the valve and endocardium. Infected tissue embolising from an infected valve on the left side of the heart may result in cerebral, renal, or more unusually, bone abscesses.

5 Guidelines to reduce the risk of this disease occurring

In the UK, guidelines are available from the British Heart Foundation in conjunction with the British Society for Antimicrobial Agents and Chemotherapy on the use of antimicrobial prophylaxis before dentistry. Prophylactic and therapeutic guidelines are available in most countries.

Although there is little evidence that the majority of cases of endocarditis are due to dental manipulation, litigation has ensued where a dentist has failed to give prophylaxis to patients known to be at risk of endocarditis.

14 INFECTION IN THE IMMUNOCOMPROMISED HOST

CASE 49

see Mims 33.8

A 43-year-old woman has chronic renal failure. She has undergone regular haemodialysis and has been on the renal transplant programme for two years. She is seen by the renal physicians because a suitable kidney has been donated that day. Baseline serological antibody tests had been performed and she is cytomegalovirus (CMV) antibody negative, varicella zoster virus antibody positive, HIV 1 and 2 antibody negative, hepatitis C virus (HCV) antibody negative, hepatitis B surface antigen (HBsAg) negative and anti-HB core negative. The donor kidney is an excellent HLA match, and the donor was HIV 1 and 2 antibody negative, HCV antibody negative, HBsAg negative, and CMV antibody positive.

A renal transplant is performed that evening and she is started on the usual immunosuppressive drug regimen in order to avert the onset of graft versus host disease (organ rejection). In addition, she is started on prophylaxis with acyclovir and cotrimoxazole to prevent herpes simplex and *Pneumocystis* infections which occur in heavily immunosuppressed patients.

Ten weeks after the successful transplant she develops a high fever, shotty lymphadenopathy, and breathlessness. On examination her temperature is 39°C, and she has shotty cervical and axillary lymphadenopathy and a rapid respiratory rate. Chest auscultation is normal as is examination of her abdomen apart from a healed scar over the site of the transplant. The results of investigations are given in Fig. 14.1.

FIG. 14.1 RESULTS OF INVESTIGATIONS

Investigation	Result
Haemoglobin	12 g/dl
White cell count	1.2×10^9 /l with a few atypical lymphocytes
Platelets	100×10^9 /l
Chest radiograph	Groundglass appearance with bilateral shadowing consistent with a pneumonitis.

Questions

1 What do you think the most likely diagnosis is?
2 How would you investigate her further?
3 The results of further investigations are shown in Fig. 14.2. How do you interpret these results?

FIG. 14.2 RESULTS OF INVESTIGATIONS

Investigation	Result
Blood gas analysis	Hypoxia (low partial pressure of oxygen)
Blood cultures, MSU, bronchoalveolar lavage, and bronchial biopsy	No bacterial growth
Heparinised blood sample	CMV DEAFF test negative
Throat swab, urine, and bronchoalveolar samples	CMV-infected cell nuclei detected, e.g. CMV DEAFF test positive
Bronchial biopsy histology	Inclusion bodies (owl's eye appearance)

4 She improves on the treatment discussed in answer 3 and makes a full recovery. What preventive measures could have been taken?

Your answers

1 Most likely diagnosis

2 Further investigation

3 Interpretation of the results of the further tests

4 Preventive measures

CASE 49

Answers

1 Most likely diagnosis

In this CMV antibody negative renal transplant recipient who receives a kidney from a CMV antibody positive donor and develops a fever, minor lymphadenopathy, and breathlessness ten weeks after transplantation, the most likely diagnosis is a primary CMV infection with dissemination to the lungs resulting in a pneumonitis. Herpes simplex pneumonitis should also be considered, although she was given acyclovir prophylaxis.

2 Further investigation

- Arterial blood gas analysis.
- Bronchoscopy and bronchoalveolar lavage (lung washings).
- Blood cultures and mid-stream urine (MSU) specimen to check for bacterial causes.
- Heparinised blood, throat swab, and urine specimens for CMV DEAFF (Detection of Early Antigenic Fluorescent Foci) testing and virus isolation in cell culture.
- If a bronchoalveolar lavage is collected this can also be used for DEAFF testing and viral isolation. Isolation may take up to 21 days to demonstrate a cytopathic effect.
  The DEAFF test is a rapid diagnostic assay in which a tissue culture monolayer grown on a coverslip is incubated overnight with potentially CMV-infected lymphocytes from the blood sample. The other specimens which may contain CMV infected cells are similarly incubated. The following day the coverslip monolayers are incubated with a cocktail of monoclonal antibodies tagged to fluorescein that are specific to the CMV early antigen gene product, and they are looked at with an ultraviolet microscope. The appearance of small green 'slipper-shaped' CMV-infected cell nuclei is characteristic of CMV infection.
- Serum specimen for CMV IgM detection, though this is not the ideal choice of test in an immunosuppressed individual who may have impaired antibody responses.

3 Interpretation of the results of the further tests

She has had a primary CMV infection that has resulted in a CMV pneumonitis. It is thought that the pathogenesis of the pneumonitis is immunopathological and it has been demonstrated that the treatment of choice is a combined approach using intravenous ganciclovir and CMV hyperimmune globulin. Ganciclovir is an antiviral drug that is myelosuppressive but is the treatment of choice for CMV infections, an alternative being foscarnet.

4 Preventive measures

- Matching the recipient and donor with respect to their CMV serological status as well as their tissue types is extremely important, but unfortunately there are instances where it is not possible to do this due to the shortage of organs for transplantation. In addition, the situation is more complicated for bone marrow transplant patients, in particular allografts, in whom CMV matching is also critical. The recipient's serological status is important in these cases because the disease is due to reactivation of CMV in a background of intense immunosuppression compared with solid organ transplants.
- Surveillance, using preservative-free heparinised blood, throat swab and urine specimens on a regular basis, using the DEAFF test for rapid diagnosis in order to monitor for CMV infection.
- Ganciclovir prophylaxis in organ recipients at risk of CMV infection.

HOSPITAL INFECTIONS

CASE 50

see Mims 33.6, 39.4

As a surgeon you are called by the nurses to see a patient who has developed a fever. Three days ago he underwent a colonic resection for carcinoma of the colon. The operation went smoothly, and he was progressing well on the ward. His past medical history before admission was unremarkable, although he is noted to be a smoker.

On examination his temperature is 37.8°C. He is slightly dyspnoeic at rest and there are a few basal crackles in his chest at both bases. His abdominal wound is dressed and you are reluctant to disturb the dressings.

Questions

1 What are the common causes of postoperative infections in patients and what steps can be taken to reduce these problems?
2 What investigations would you order?
3 How would you treat him?

Notes for revision

Your answers

1 Common causes of postoperative infections in patients and steps to reduce these problems

2 Investigations

3 Treatment

CASE 50

Answers

1 Common causes of postoperative infections in patients and steps to reduce these problems

The most common cause of a postoperative pyrexia is a wound infection. Other causes of pyrexia include chest and urinary infections. Chest infections are particularly common after abdominal surgery because the patient is in pain and finds coughing difficult. Urinary infections are often a result of catheterisation. Non-infectious causes of postoperative pyrexia include deep venous thrombosis.

Surgical wound infections are substantially reduced by giving prophylactic antibiotics which should be effective against the most common pathogens responsible for infection in that type of surgery.

2 Investigations

It is important that the wound dressing is removed in order to examine the wound and a swab is taken. Sputum culture and urine culture should also be sent. A chest radiograph is needed if there is clinical evidence of a chest infection.

This man's wound is red and discharging small amounts of pus at the lower end and a wound swab grows *Staphylococcus aureus*.

3 Treatment

Initially he would be treated with flucloxacillin. The laboratory will have the results of antibiotic sensitivity testing the following day. Methicillin is used in the laboratory to detect flucloxacillin resistance. The organism is resistant to flucloxacillin and is referred to as a Methicillin Resistant Staphylococcus Aureus or MRSA strain.

The patient should be source isolated in a side-room and staff should be made aware of the risks of carrying the organism on their hands. *Staph. aureus* is carried on a variety of sites on the body, including the nose, hair, axillae, wrists and hands, and the perineum. Swabs should be collected from these sites in this patient to check for carriage.

The carriage rate is higher in hospitals than outside in the community. MRSA ward outbreaks may occur, especially as the organism survives in dry environments. In this case, the most likely source of the MRSA is the patient's skin or nose.

The following measures should be taken in order to reduce the chance of the MRSA spreading: these include source isolating the patient, careful wound dressing technique and good hand washing technique by any member of staff attending him. In addition, he should be treated with a glycopeptide antibiotic, either vancomycin or teicoplanin. If vancomycin is used, the serum levels must be monitored.

F

Fifth's disease (parvovirus B19) 74
Flucloxacillin 18, 76, 78, 92
Fluconazole 60
5-Fluorocytosine 60
Foreign body, inhaled 10
Foscarnet 12
Frenal ulcer 16
Fusidic acid 76, 78

G

Gammabenzene hexachloride 36
Ganciclovir 12, 90
Gangrene 75–76
Gas gangrene 76
Gastritis 43–44
Gastroenteritis, viral 39–40
Gentamicin 41–42, 44, 52, 68, 76
German measles (rubella) 70, 74
Glandular fever 80
Glue ear 10
Gonorrhoea 34, 78
Graft versus host disease 89
Group A streptococci 54, 72
Group B streptococci 52

H

H$_2$ antagonists 44
Haemophilus influenzae 10, 16, 47, 62
    capsular type b (Hib) 10
Heart valve, prosthetic 87–88
Helicobacter pylori 44
Hepatitis B infection 38
Herpes simplex virus
    cervical 30
    encephalitis 58
    meningitis 56
    myocarditis 70
Heterophile antibody 80
HIV
    antibody screening 32
    central nervous system infection 59–60
    Pneumocystis carinii pneumonia 32
Human herpes virus 6 (HHV6) 74

I

Immunisation
    hepatitis B 38
    Hib 10
    influenza 18
    meningococcal 62
    pertussis 16
    pneumococcal 22
Immunosuppression 89–90
Infectious mononucleosis (glandular fever) 80
Influenza viruses 18, 20, 70
Insect bites 71–72
Isoniazid 24

J

Jarisch–Herxheimer reaction 36
Joint infection 77–78

L

Lactose intolerance/malabsorption 40
Legionella pneumophila 14
Leptospirosis 86
Lice, pubic 36
Listeria monocytogenes 52, 68
Lumbar puncture 55
Lymphadenopathy
    cervical 79
    immunosuppression 89–90
Lymphoma, gastric 44

M

Malaria 50, 82
Malathion 36
Mastoiditis 10
Measles 70, 74
Meningitis
    aseptic (viral) 56
    bacterial 68
    meningococcal 62
    pneumococcal 64
Methicillin-resistant *Staph. aureus* (MRSA) 54, 92
Methylprednisolone 32
Metronidazole 30, 41–42, 44, 48, 66, 76
Monoarthritis, acute 77–78
Moraxella catarrhalis 10
Mumps 56, 58, 70
Mycobacterium tuberculosis 12, 24, 68
Mycoplasma spp. 18
    M. pneumoniae 13–14
Myocarditis, viral 70

N

Neisseria gonorrhoeae 30, 34, 78
Neisseria meningitidis 62
Neonatal infection 52, 68
Nitrofurantoin 28

O

Obstruction, respiratory 10
Omeprazole 44
Osteomyelitis, acute 76
Otitis media 10, 66

P

Parainfluenza viruses 20
Parasites
    malarial 82
    ova and cysts, identification 46
Particle agglutination test 14
Parvovirus B19 74
Penicillin 34, 78

Pentamidine 32
Pericarditis, relapsing 70
Peritonitis 41–42
Pertussis 16
Photophobia 55, 63
Phthirus pubis 36
Pneumocystis carinii pneumonia 32
Pneumonia
    atypical 13–14
    bronchopneumonia 16
    lobar 22
    Pneumocystis carinii 32
Pneumonitis 90
Polio 70
Postoperative infection 92
Pregnancy
    chickenpox 71–72
    Listeria monocytogenes 68
    urinary tract infection 27–28
Probenecid 36
Procaine penicillin 36
Prophylactic antibiotics 88, 92
Prostatic hypertrophy, benign 28
Pseudomembranous colitis 48
Pyelonephritis 28
Pyrexia of unknown origin 49–50, 83–84, 91–92

Q

Q fever (*Coxiella burnetii*) 14, 18

R

Rabies 70
Rapid MicroAgglutination Test (RMAT) 14
Renal failure 54
Renal transplantation 89–90
Respiratory synctial virus (RSV) 19–20
Retinitis 11–12
Reverse passive haemagglutination (RPHA) test 38
Rheumatic valve disease 88
Ribavirin 20
Rifampicin 24, 62, 84
Roseola infantum (exanthema subitum) 74
Rotavirus infection 39–40
Rubella 70, 74

S

Salmonella typhi 50
Sarcoptes scabei 36
Scabies 35–36
Septicaemia
    infants 62
    newborn 52
Shigella spp. 46
Sickle cell disease 21–22
Space-occupying lesions 66
Splenectomy 22

Splenomegaly 79
Staphylococci, coagulase-negative 88
Staphylococcus aureus 10, 18, 54, 66, 76, 78, 88, 92
    methicillin-resistant 54, 92
Streptococci
    group A 54, 72
    group B 52
    non group A beta haemolytic 78
    S. milleri 44, 66
    S. pneumoniae 10, 22, 62, 68, 78
    S. viridans 88
Subarachnoid haemorrhage 58, 68
Subdural haematoma 58, 68
Sugar fermentation tests 34
Super antigens 54
Syphilis, tertiary 35–36

T

Tabes dorsalis 36
Teicoplanin 22, 92
Tetracycline 14
Toxic shock syndrome 54
Toxocara canis/catis 12
Toxoplasma gondii 12
Trauma, central nervous system 66
Trichomonas vaginalis 30
Tuberculosis 50
    pulmonary 24
Typhoid 50, 82

U

^{13}C Urea breath test 44
Ureaplasma urealyticum 34
Urethritis 34
Urinary tract infection 92
    acute urinary retention 27–28
    infants 26
    pregnancy 27–28
Urinary retention, acute 27–28

V

Vaccination *see* Immunisation
Vaginal discharge 29–30
Vancomycin 22, 48, 92
Varicella zoster virus 72
Vesico-ureteric reflux 26
Viral haemorrhagic fever 82

W

Whooping cough (pertussis) 16
Wound infection 92

Z

Zoster immune globulin 72